Gastrointestinal Anatomy an

We dedicate this book to our teachers and students, and to our families, especially our wives: Enid and Doreen, this book is for you with our undying gratitude for your boundless love and support.

Gastrointestinal Anatomy and Physiology

The Essentials

EDITED BY

John F. Reinus, MD

Chief of Clinical Hepatology
Division of Gastroenterology and Liver Diseases
Montefiore Medical Center
Professor of Clinical Medicine
The Albert Einstein College of Medicine
Bronx, NY, USA

Douglas Simon, MD, FACG

Chief of Gastroenterology and Hepatology
Jacobi Medical Center
Professor of Clinical Medicine
The Albert Einstein College of Medicine
Bronx, NY, USA

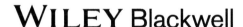

Library of Congress Cataloging-in-Publication Data

Gastrointestinal anatomy and physiology : the essentials / edited by John F. Reinus, Douglas Simon.
    p. ; cm.
    Includes bibliographical references and index.
    ISBN 978-0-470-67484-0 (pbk. : alk. paper)
I. Reinus, John, editor of compilation.   II. Simon, Douglas, 1956– editor of compilation.   [DNLM:
1. Digestive System–anatomy & histology.   2. Digestive System Physiological Phenomena.   WI 101]
    QP145
    612.3–dc23
                                    2013034304
A catalogue record for this book is available from the British Library.

Wiley also publishes its books in a variety of electronic formats. Some content that appears in print may not
be available in electronic books.

Cover image: © Dream Designs Image ID: 97229036
Cover design by Garth Stewart

Set in 9.5/13pt Meridien by SPi Publisher Services, Pondicherry, India

1   2014

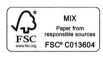

Contents

Contributors

Darren Brenner, MD
Assistant Professor of Medicine
Division of Gastroenterology
Northwestern University Feinberg School of Medicine
Chicago, IL, USA

John Del Valle, MD
Professor and Senior Associate Chair of Medicine
Department of Internal Medicine
Division of Gastroenterology
University of Michigan Medical Center
Ann Arbor, MI, USA

Lawrence S. Friedman, MD
Professor of Medicine
Harvard Medical School
Professor of Medicine
Tufts University School of Medicine
Assistant Chief of Medicine
Massachusetts General Hospital
Boston, MA, USA
The Anton R. Fried, MD, Chair
Department of Medicine
Newton-Wellesley Hospital
Newton, MA, USA

D. Neil Granger, PhD
Boyd Professor & Head
Department of Molecular & Cellular Physiology
LSU Health Sciences Center
Shreveport, LA, USA

James H. Grendell, MD
Professor of Medicine
School of Medicine
State University of New York at Stony Brook
Stony Brook, NY, USA
Chief, Division of Gastroenterology, Hepatology & Nutrition
Winthrop University Hospital
Mineola, NY, USA

Ikuo Hirano, MD
Professor of Medicine
Fellowship Program Director
Division of Gastroenterology
Northwestern University Feinberg School of Medicine
Chicago, IL, USA

Peter R. Kvietys, PhD
Professor of Physiology
College of Medicine
Alfaisal University
Riyadh, Saudi Arabia

Michelle T. Long, MD
Fellow, Division of Gastroenterology
Boston University School of Medicine and
Boston Medical Center
Boston, MA, USA

Elizabeth A. Montgomery, MD
Professor of Pathology, Oncology, and Orthopedic Surgery
Department of Pathology
Johns Hopkins Hospital
Baltimore, MD, USA

Scott E. Plevy, MD
Associate Professor
Departments of Medicine, Microbiology and Immunology
University of North Carolina School of Medicine
Chapel Hill, NC, USA

Lawrence R. Schiller, MD
Professor of Medicine
Dallas Campus, Texas A&M College of Medicine
Attending Physician
Digestive Health Associates of Texas
Program Director
Gastroenterology Fellowship
Baylor University Medical Center
Dallas, TX, USA

Mitchell L. Schubert, MD
Professor of Medicine and Physiology
Virginia Commonwealth University's Medical College of Virginia
Chief, Division of Gastroenterology
McGuire Veterans Affairs Medical Center
Richmond, VA, USA

Shehzad Z. Sheikh, MD, PhD
Assistant Professor of Medicine
Division of Gastroenterology and Hepatology
University of North Carolina School of Medicine
Chapel Hill, NC, USA

Allan W. Wolkoff, MD
The Herman Lopata Chair in Liver Disease Research
Professor of Medicine and Anatomy and Structural Biology
Associate Chair of Medicine for Research
Chief, Division of Gastroenterology and Liver Diseases
Director, Marion Bessin Liver Research Center
Albert Einstein College of Medicine and Montefiore Medical Center
Bronx, NY, USA

Laura D. Wood, MD, PhD
Assistant Professor of Pathology and Oncology
Department of Pathology
Johns Hopkins Hospital
Baltimore, MD, USA

Preface

A relatively detailed understanding of normal organ structure and function is essential to adequately evaluate, diagnose, and manage disease. The American Board of Internal Medicine has endorsed this proposition by including questions about the normal anatomy and physiology of digestive organs in the Gastroenterology Certification Examination. According to a statement published by the Board, approximately 10% of the Certification Examination questions test knowledge of these subjects.

Many years ago, during our training, we had our first discussion of how best to learn about gastrointestinal anatomy and physiology. Predominantly regional organization made it difficult to acquire an overall understanding of many important topics by studying some standard texts: in these books, conceptually related information about microscopic anatomy, motility, absorption and secretion, and of other topics was divided among chapters principally devoted to major organs, for example, the stomach or the small bowel. In addition, the overwhelming quantity of information in reference works made finding and selecting the details that were relevant to clinical practice a near-impossible task, at least from the point of view of two novice practitioners.

Several years later, we were able to persuade the members of the Educational Affairs Committee of the American College of Gastroenterology to allow us to create a review course dedicated exclusively to the subjects of normal gastrointestinal structure and function. Until its recent discontinuation, this course was offered every other year at the College's annual meeting in conjunction with its regular board review. Hundreds of gastroenterologists have benefited from the excellent presentations made at the course by many of the same individuals who have contributed chapters to this book.

It is, therefore, with great pleasure that we have seized the opportunity offered us by the people at Wiley to address in book form the subject of basic gastrointestinal structure and function. Our intention is to create a review from the perspective of what is needed to practice clinical gastroenterology and to present it in chapters devoted to specific topics in anatomy and physiology. We hope you enjoy it.

John F. Reinus and Douglas Simon
The Albert Einstein College of Medicine

About the companion website

Gastrointestinal anatomy and physiology has its own resources website:

www.wiley.com/go/reinus/gastro/anatomy

The website includes all figures from the book

CHAPTER 1

Structure and innervation of hollow viscera

Laura D. Wood & Elizabeth A. Montgomery
Department of Pathology, Johns Hopkins Hospital, Baltimore, MD, USA

The tubular gastrointestinal (GI) tract consists of hollow organs composed of distinct tissue layers: mucosa, submucosa, muscularis propria, and serosa or adventitia. The mucosa of each GI organ has a unique cellular structure, whereas the other layers are similar throughout the GI tract. Innervation of the hollow viscera consists of postsynaptic sympathetic and presynaptic parasympathetic neurons with parasympathetic ganglion cells present in the myenteric (Auerbach's) and submucosal (Meissner's) plexi. It is important to note that there is more lymphoid tissue (mucosa-associated lymphoid tissue) in the GI tract than there is in all the rest of the body combined.

The mucosa

The mucosa is the innermost layer of the GI tract; its function will be discussed in detail in the succeeding text. The mucosa has three components:
1 The epithelium, which has protective and secretory or absorptive properties.
2 The lamina propria, a loose connective tissue zone supporting the avascular epithelium. In the esophagus, stomach, and small intestine, but not the colorectum, the lamina propria has many lymphatics, allowing mucosal tumors to easily invade the lymphatics of the upper GI tract. In the upper GI tract, there are fewer immune cells (lymphoid and plasma cells) in the lamina propria than there are in the lamina propria of the small bowel and colon.
3 The muscularis mucosae, a narrow double layer of inner circular and outer longitudinal smooth muscle separating the mucosa from the submucosa. The muscularis mucosae resembles the muscularis propria but in miniature.

Gastrointestinal Anatomy and Physiology: The Essentials, First Edition. Edited by John F. Reinus and Douglas Simon.
© 2014 John Wiley & Sons, Ltd. Published 2014 by John Wiley & Sons, Ltd.
www.wiley.com/go/reinus/gastro/anatomy

The submucosa

The submucosa is composed of connective tissue and contains Meissner's nerve plexus as well as large-caliber blood vessels.

The muscularis propria

The muscularis propria gives structural strength to the hollow viscera. It is composed of an inner circular and outer longitudinal layer of smooth muscle. Between these layers is Auerbach's nerve plexus.

Serosa or adventitia

The outermost layer of the GI tract is either a serosa or an adventitia. The latter is distinguished by its lack of a mesothelial membrane lining.

Parasympathetic ganglion cells are found in Meissner's and Auerbach's nerve plexi. The submucosal Meissner's plexi also contain neuronal cell bodies of the intrinsic sympathetic nerve system that function on the local area of the gut. These are the neurons that have chemoreceptors and mechanoreceptors. They synapse on both other ganglion cells and on muscle and secretory cells.

Esophagus

The esophagus is about 25 cm in length and consists of a cervical and upper-, mid-, and lower-thoracic segments. It is physiologically constricted by the cricoid cartilage, the aortic arch, the left atrium, and the diaphragm. The esophagus is unique among the hollow viscera in that it has skeletal (voluntary) muscle, which surrounds its upper portions. The vagus nerve provides the esophagus with parasympathetic innervation, whereas its sympathetic innervation is from the cervical and paravertebral ganglia.

Histologically, the squamous mucosa of the esophagus is heaped up in folds (Figure 1.1a and b). The mitotically active basal layer matures completely into a surface layer containing tonofilaments within 10 days. The basal layer comprises about 15% of the esophageal epithelial thickness. The cells become flatter and more eosinophilic as they approach the surface. The normal esophageal epithelium lacks a granular layer (present in skin) and does not keratinize. A small number of T lymphocytes are normally present in the epithelium.

Beneath the esophageal epithelium is the lamina propria, which contains numerous small capillary-sized blood vessels and lymphatics as well as elastic fibers. The esophageal lamina propria has very few lymphocytes and essentially no

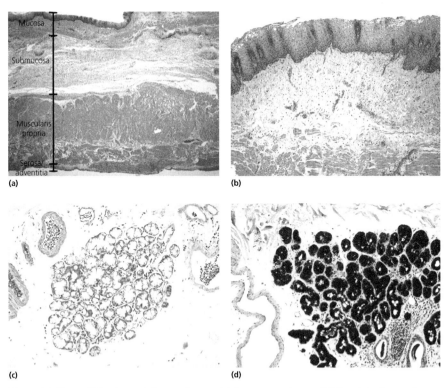

Figure 1.1 Normal histology of the esophagus. (a) Low-power image (H&E stain) of normal esophagus illustrating the characteristic layers of the wall – mucosa, submucosa, muscularis propria, and adventitia/serosa. A submucosal gland can be seen at the right side of the image. (b) Medium-power image (H&E stain) of the esophageal mucosa, with stratified squamous epithelium, lamina propria, and muscularis mucosae. Note the rich vascularity in the lamina propria. (c) High-power image (H&E stain) of an esophageal submucosal gland. (d) High-power image (PAS-AB stain) of an esophageal submucosal gland with characteristic dark blue color.

eosinophils or plasma cells. The lymphovascular network of the lamina propria facilitates spread of invading cancers, as do similar networks in the stomach and small intestine (but not the colon).

The muscularis mucosae of the esophagus is a slender layer that rapidly thickens in response to injury; resultant reduplication of this layer may make cancer staging difficult. Normally, the smooth muscle fibers of the muscularis mucosae are mostly longitudinal in orientation. There is no skeletal muscle in the esophageal muscularis mucosae (in contrast to the esophageal muscularis propria which contains skeletal muscle fibers). In the upper esophagus, the muscularis mucosae blends with the fibrous membrane of the hypopharynx, whereas in the lower esophagus, it merges with the muscularis mucosae of the stomach.

The submucosa of the esophagus is composed of loose connective tissue with abundant elastic fibers, a rich lymphovascular network that has well-developed venous plexi, scattered ganglion cells, and nerve fibers of Meissner's plexus.

The esophageal submucosa also contains glands (Figure 1.1c and d). These glands are composed of mucin-producing cells that are deeply alcianophilic on periodic acid–Schiff–Alcian blue (PAS-AB) staining. They may undergo various types of metaplasia in response to injury. Ducts lined by cuboidal epithelium convey mucus secreted by the glands to the luminal surface of the esophagus where it lubricates the passage of food.

The esophageal muscularis propria is composed of striated muscle in the upper esophagus, smooth muscle in the lower esophagus, and a mixture of the two in between. The amounts of smooth and striated muscle are said to become equal about 5 cm below the esophageal–pharyngeal junction. There is a well-developed neural plexus (Auerbach's plexus) between the inner circular and outer longitudinal muscle layers. The inner circular layer of the lower esophagus, or lower esophageal sphincter (LES), contracts or relaxes in response to gastrin or secretin. There are no specific histologic features that distinguish the LES from the rest of the muscularis propria.

The esophagus has an adventitia, a layer of coarse connective tissue that connects the esophagus to adjoining structures, in particular the mediastinum. The adventitia contains thick nerves, blood vessels, and lymphatics.

Stomach

The stomach has four parts, each with different mucosal features: the cardia (most proximal), fundus, body, and antrum (most distal). The cardia and antrum are histologically similar and have the function of protecting the esophagus (cardia) or duodenum (antrum) from the acid and enzymes present in the rest of the organ. The cardia expands, and may even be acquired, as a result of acid injury and other insults in the region of the gastroesophageal junction [1–5]. The stomach receives sympathetic innervation from the celiac plexus and parasympathetic innervation from the vagus nerve.

The luminal surface of the empty stomach has thick longitudinal folds, or rugae, with tiny surface invaginations called gastric pits, which allow gastric glandular secretions to reach the mucosal surface. These glands, regardless of their location in the stomach, have an isthmus, neck, and base and are complex, convoluted structures that are difficult to visualize in three dimensions based on their microscopic appearance in two dimensions (Figure 1.2a and b). The entire surface of the stomach, including the gastric pits, is lined by foveolar cells that secrete neutral mucin and appear pink on PAS stain (Figure 1.2c and d).

The glands of the gastric body and fundus are similar in structure. The most common cell type of the gland isthmus is the mucous neck cell. These cells also are found in the neck where parietal (oxyntic) cells are most numerous. The chief cell is found at the base of the gland. The areas of the gland with parietal and chief cells do not stain with PAS-AB because they do not contain mucin (Figure 1.2d).

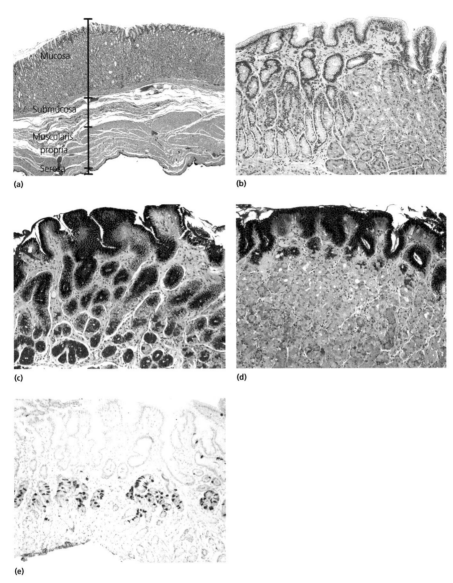

(a)

(b)

(c)

(d)

(e)

Figure 1.2 Normal histology of the stomach. (a) Low-power image (H&E stain) of normal stomach (body) illustrating the characteristic layers of the wall – mucosa, submucosa, muscularis propria, and serosa. (b) Medium-power image (H&E stain) of transitional gastric epithelium. On the right, oxyntic epithelium consists of surface foveolar cells overlying oxyntic glands with parietal and chief cells. On the left, antral epithelium consists of foveolar cells overlying mucin-producing antral glands. (c) Medium-power image (PAS-AB stain) of antral epithelium, illustrating the bright pink staining of both the foveolar cells and the antral glands. (d) Medium-power image (PAS-AB) stain of oxyntic epithelium, with bright pink staining of foveolar cells but lack of staining in the parietal and chief cells of the oxyntic glands. (e) Antral mucosa (gastrin immunohistochemical stain), illustrating the presence of gastrin-producing G cells in the antral glands. Gastrin immunohistochemical stain is negative in oxyntic mucosa and in cardiac mucosa.

Endocrine cells are found in the deep isthmus toward the gland base. The cardiac and antral glands are neutral mucin-producing glands that stain pink with PAS-AB (Figure 1.2c). The cardia and antrum are very similar histologically, but the antrum contains G cells, whereas the cardia does not (Figure 1.2e).

The G cells of the antrum secrete gastrin, which stimulates enterochromaffin-like cells of the gastric body and fundus to secrete histamine. Histamine in turn stimulates acid secretion by parietal cells of the gastric body and fundus. In addition, gastrin has a trophic effect on parietal cells. The antrum also contains D cells that secrete somatostatin, which inhibits G-cell gastrin secretion. All these endocrine interactions are important in disease states. For example, in autoimmune gastritis, patients have immune damage to parietal cells that results in hypergastrinemia, because antral G cells secrete excess gastrin in an attempt to stimulate acid production. Autoimmune damage to parietal cells, which produce intrinsic factor, results in pernicious anemia.

The lamina propria of the stomach contains small numbers of plasma cells, eosinophils, mast cells, and lymphocytes. Lymphatics and blood vessels are less numerous than they are in the lamina propria of the esophagus. Scattered lymphoid aggregates are present. Bacteria are absent from normal gastric mucosa, whereas mucosal bacteria are seen in the esophagus and ileocolon.

The muscularis mucosae of the stomach contains an inner circular and outer longitudinal layer of smooth muscle. In some instances, a third slim circular layer is present.

The submucosa of the stomach is formed of connective tissue with elastic fibers and has prominent blood vessels, as does the lamina propria of other parts of the tubular GI tract. Meissner's plexus is found in the gastric submucosa.

The gastric muscularis propria consists of three fairly indistinct layers: an inner oblique, middle circular, and outer longitudinal layer. The layers are somewhat randomly oriented and may be absent or poorly developed in some areas. This random arrangement of muscle fibers is typical of hollow organs that expel their contents (e.g., uterus, urinary bladder, gallbladder). The muscularis propria contains Auerbach's plexus and ganglion cells. Interstitial cells of Cajal (ICCs), also called "pacemaker" cells, can be readily identified in the muscularis propria using immunolabeling with antibodies directed against CD117 (c-kit protein).

The stomach is encased by a serosa that is composed of connective tissue and a lining of flat-to-cuboidal peritoneal cells, a unique type of modified epithelial cell. This contrasts with the connective tissue covering the esophagus.

Small bowel

The small bowel is divided into three major sections. The duodenum extends from the gastric pylorus to the ligament of Treitz and is formed sequentially of a bulb and descending, horizontal, and ascending portions. The duodenum is

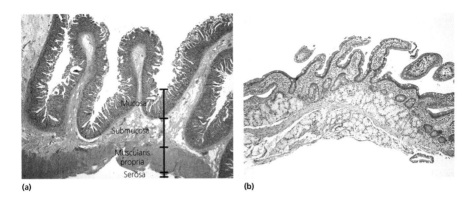

(a)

(b)

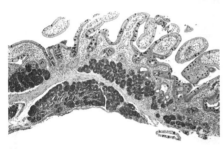

(c)

Figure 1.3 Normal histology of the small bowel. (a) Low-power image (H&E stain) of normal small bowel with plicae circulares and epithelial villi. The small bowel contains the same layers as the other organs of the tubular GI tract – mucosa, submucosa, muscularis propria, and serosa. (b) Medium-power image (H&E stain) of the duodenal mucosa and submucosa, illustrating the presence of Brunner's glands in the lamina propria and submucosa. Strictly speaking, Brunner's glands should be restricted to the submucosa, but most adult patients have Brunner's glands in the duodenal lamina propria, presumably a reparative change. (c) Medium-power image (PAS-AB stain) of the duodenal mucosa and submucosa, illustrating the bright pink staining of Brunner's glands. Note that the goblet cells contain alcianophilic purple-colored mucin, whereas the absorptive cells lack mucin.

mostly retroperitoneal, whereas the jejunum and ileum are intraperitoneal. The jejunum is distal to the ligament of Treitz and consists, somewhat arbitrarily, of the proximal third of the intraperitoneal small bowel. The jejunum narrows into the ileum, which is formed by the distal two-thirds of the intraperitoneal small bowel and joins the colon at the ileocecal valve. These sections of the small bowel receive parasympathetic innervation from the vagus nerves and sympathetic innervation from the celiac plexus.

Like the esophagus and stomach, the small bowel wall consists of layers: mucosa (epithelium, lamina propria, muscularis mucosae), submucosa, muscularis propria, and serosa or adventitia (Figure 1.3a). The unique gross and microscopic anatomy of the small bowel reflects its principal function, absorption of nutrients. Macroscopic plicae circulares and microscopic villous projections of the epithelium and lamina propria give a tube 6–7-m long an absorptive surface of 200–500 m². Villi are broad in the duodenum and ileum and are long and thin in the jejunum. In between villi, the epithelium forms invaginations, or glands, referred to as "crypts of Lieberkühn." The villus-to-crypt height ratio is quite variable throughout the small bowel, ranging from 2–3:1 in the proximal duodenum to 4–5:1 in the jejunum.

Small bowel villi and crypts are lined mainly by absorptive cells that have a microvillus brush border consisting of numerous cytoplasmic projections that further expand the enterocyte's absorptive surface. Absorptive cells of the small bowel lack mucin, including the neutral mucin found in the foveolar cells of the stomach [6]. Although most epithelial cells are absorptive, the epithelium also contains scattered goblet cells with large vacuoles of acid mucin. There also are scattered Paneth cells in the crypts of the small bowel, with basal nuclei and red granular apical cytoplasm, as well as endocrine cells with apical nuclei and granular basal cytoplasm. These two cell types have a similar appearance but opposite orientation relative to the basement membrane, and the granules of endocrine cells are smaller than those of Paneth cells. Paneth cells have large eosinophilic granules containing growth factors and antimicrobial proteins, while endocrine cells have fine granules containing a variety of peptides and bioactive compounds.

The lamina propria of the small bowel contains numerous lymphocytes and plasma cells (primarily IgA-secreting) as well as scattered eosinophils. Capillaries and lacteals, blindly ending lymphatic vessels that absorb chylomicrons, are found in the lamina propria at the tips of the villi. The lamina propria of the villi also contains delicate strands of smooth muscle.

The small bowel muscularis mucosae consists of slim inner circular and outer longitudinal layers of smooth muscle. The crypt bases reach the top of the muscularis mucosae.

The small bowel submucosa is composed of loose connective tissue and contains large-caliber vessels and Meissner's nerve plexus of both parasympathetic ganglion cells and sympathetic neurons. In the duodenum, the submucosa is the site of Brunner's glands, mucin-producing glands that are unique to the duodenum and contain neutral mucin (Figure 1.3b and c). The submucosa also contains lymphoid aggregates, often with germinal centers. These lymphoid aggregates, or Peyer's patches (PPs), are present throughout the small bowel but are most numerous in the ileum. While they have a linear orientation in the duodenum and jejunum, they are arrayed circumferentially in the ileum where they create a potential for intussusception if they undergo hypertrophy. Numerous intraepithelial lymphocytes (IELs) are present in the epithelium overlying the PPs; these lymphocytes communicate with the rest of the lymphoid compartment through specialized epithelial cells known as M cells.

The muscularis propria is a thick double layer of inner circular and outer longitudinal muscle that generates the propulsive action of the bowel wall and is the source of most of its tensile strength. Auerbach's nerve plexus of parasympathetic ganglion cells is located between the muscle layers.

The outermost layer of the intraperitoneal small bowel (jejunum and ileum) is serosa. The retroperitoneal small bowel (duodenum) is covered by mesothelium on its anterior surface only; the posterior surface is covered by loose connective tissue, so the duodenum has an anterior serosa and a posterior adventitia.

Colon and rectum

The colon has several anatomically distinct parts: The cecum and ascending colon are fixed by mesentery to the posterior right abdominal wall; only their anterior surfaces are covered by peritoneal mesothelium. The transverse colon is suspended in the abdominal cavity by the lesser omentum and is completely covered by serosa. The descending colon is adherent to the posterior left abdominal wall and, like the ascending colon, only has a peritoneal membrane on its anterior surface. The sigmoid colon is the only part of the colon suspended entirely by mesentery and is therefore completely covered by serosa. The rectum is adherent to the posterior abdominal wall. The colon receives parasympathetic innervation from the vagus nerve proximally and pelvic splanchnic nerves distally. Its sympathetic innervation comes from the superior and inferior mesenteric plexi.

Like the rest of the hollow viscera, the colon has a layered bowel wall with a mucosa (epithelium, lamina propria, muscularis mucosae), submucosa, muscularis propria, and serosa or adventitia (Figure 1.4a). Because the function of the colon is to absorb water and electrolytes, its mucosal architecture is different from that of the small bowel. Grossly, the colon has transverse mucosal folds, plicae semilunares, with haustral sacs between the folds. The colonic mucosa, unlike the small bowel mucosa, is mostly flat, although it may have smooth undulations known as anthemic folds. The colon epithelium does not have villi; it has straight invaginations called crypts, which line up like "test tubes in a rack" (Figure 1.4b). The crypt epithelium mostly consists of goblet cells, each with a single large mucin vacuole, but a few absorptive cells also are present [7]. Scattered IELs normally are found throughout the colon [8]. In the bases of the crypts, there are precursor cells as well as endocrine cells that exhibit the same morphology as endocrine cells in the small intestine. Paneth cells, with basal nuclei and apical red granular cytoplasm like those in the small intestine, normally are present in the crypt bases of the ascending and transverse colons but are absent from the crypts of the normal descending and sigmoid colons.

The colonic lamina propria contains a mixture of lymphocytes, plasma cells, and eosinophils. Inflammatory cells are more abundant in the lamina propria of the ascending colon than in that of the descending colon; therefore, knowledge of biopsy location is necessary to accurately interpret signs of

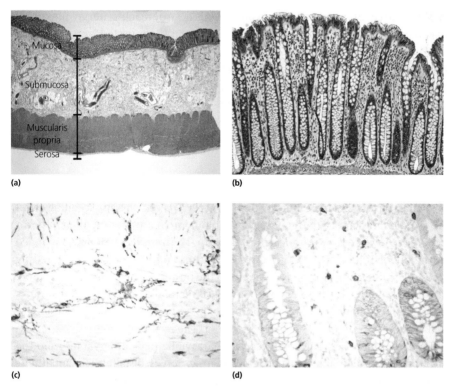

Figure 1.4 Normal histology of the colon. (a) Low-power image (H&E stain) of normal colon illustrating the characteristic layers – mucosa, submucosa, muscularis propria, and serosa. Large vessels are apparent in the submucosa but not the lamina propria. (b) Medium-power image (H&E stain) of normal colonic mucosa, with regular crypts lined by mucin-producing goblet cells arranged like "test tubes in a rack" and abuting on the muscularis mucosae. (c) Muscularis propria of the colon (CD117 immunohistochemical stain), illustrating the presence of numerous ICCs scattered throughout the muscularis propria. (d) Lamina propria of the colon (CD117 immunohistochemical stain), illustrating the (normal) presence of mast cells in the lamina propria – these cells should not be confused with ICCs, which are also positive for CD117.

inflammation. Importantly, the lamina propria of the colon lacks lymphatic vessels, a critical point in the staging of invading neoplasms. Whereas neoplasms invading the lamina propria of other parts of the GI tract may metastasize, those that penetrate the colonic lamina propria are considered in situ lesions (intramucosal carcinoma), as the lack of lymphatics reduces the likelihood of metastasis.

Beneath the lamina propria is the slender colonic muscularis mucosae, with inner circular and outer longitudinal layers of smooth muscle. In the normal colon, the crypt bases line up evenly along the top of the muscularis mucosae.

The submucosa of the colon is composed of loose connective tissue and contains large-caliber vessels as well as Meissner's nerve plexus of parasympathetic ganglion cells and sympathetic neurons.

The colonic muscularis propria has inner circular and outer longitudinal muscle layers that, as in the rest of the luminal gut, generate propulsive action and are a source of tensile strength. Auerbach's nerve plexus of parasympathetic ganglion cells is located between the layers and includes ICCs, also called pacemaker cells (Figure 1.4c). The muscularis propria of the colon is unique in that the circular muscle is continuous throughout the length and circumference of the colon, whereas the outer longitudinal layer is discontinuous. The longitudinal smooth muscle is arrayed in three symmetrically positioned bundles, the tenia coli. One is at the site of the colon's mesenteric attachment (tenia mesocolica), another is at the site of the attachment of the greater omentum to the transverse colon (tenia omentalis), and a third band is "free" (tenia libera). Polypoid collections of adipose tissue, the epiploic appendages, project from the outer surface of the colon over the two antimesenteric tenia. Blood vessels enter the bowel wall on either side of the tenia mesocolica and on the mesenteric sides of the tenia omentalis and the tenia libera. These sites of entry create weak points in the bowel wall where colonic diverticula may develop.

The proximal half of the rectum is within the abdominal cavity and is covered by peritoneum; the distal half is embedded in the soft tissue of the pelvis and lacks a peritoneal covering. This point is crucial to the evaluation of surgical specimens, as the external surface of the distal rectum represents a true surgical margin rather than a peritonealized surface. In the distal rectum, the teniae coli merge to once again form a continuous layer of longitudinal smooth muscle.

Although the rectal mucosa has the same basic components as do the mucosal surfaces of the rest of the colon, it also has some unique features. The rectal crypts are often shorter, with wider and less regular spacing. These crypts may be less numerous and have irregular shapes.

The lamina propria of the rectum is often more cellular than that of the descending and sigmoid colons, with lymphocytes, plasma cells, neutrophils, and mucoprotein-containing histiocytes (muciphages). Mild fibrosis also may be seen.

Anus

Where the bowel joins the anal canal, the transverse plicae semilunares are replaced by longitudinal anal columns. These columns terminate in the anal valves, which contain the anal sinuses, mucosal recesses into which the mucin-producing anal glands empty. This circumferential ring of anal valves is also known as the dentate line.

The anal mucosa can be divided into three regions based on the characteristics of its epithelial lining (Figure 1.5a). There is, however, considerable individual

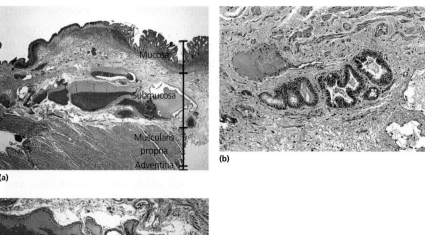

(a)

(b)

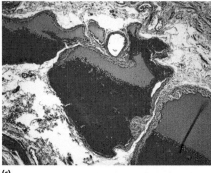

(c)

Figure 1.5 Normal histology of the anus. (a) Low-power image (H&E stain) of anus with dilated hemorrhoidal blood vessels in the submucosa. The mucosa consists of colonic (right), transitional (center), and squamous (left) regions. The anus consists of the characteristic layers, with an adventitia due to its retroperitoneal location. (b) High-power image (H&E stain) of a submucosal anal gland. (c) Medium-power image (H&E stain) of dilated hemorrhoidal vessels in the submucosa of the anus.

variation in the extent of these epithelial areas. Proximally, the anal epithelium is similar to the columnar epithelium of the rectum and has crypts lined mostly by goblet cells. Distally, the anus has a nonkeratinizing stratified squamous epithelium that becomes keratinized skin with adnexal structures distal to the anal verge. The transition from columnar to squamous epithelia, usually located in the region of the dentate line, is quite variable in appearance. In some cases, columnar rectal epithelium is located directly adjacent to stratified squamous epithelium with little if any intervening transitional epithelium. In other cases, the columnar and squamous epithelia are separated by a transitional epithelium consisting of four to nine layers of stratified cuboidal cells that are neither squamous nor columnar (with a similar morphology to the transitional epithelium of the urinary bladder).

In all three regions, the characteristic layers of the tubular gut underlie the anal epithelium. The anal submucosa, muscularis mucosae, and lamina propria are similar to those elsewhere in the GI tract, with unique anal glands in the submucosa (Figure 1.5b). In addition, the submucosa of the anus frequently contains dilated hemorrhoidal blood vessels (Figure 1.5c).

Due to its role in regulation of defecation, the musculature of the anus (including the muscularis propria) forms unique sphincters. The smooth muscle of the anal muscularis propria forms the involuntarily controlled internal anal sphincter, while anorectal skeletal muscle forms the voluntarily controlled external anal sphincter. The parasympathetic innervation of the anus comes from the pelvic splanchnic nerves, and the sympathetic innervation comes from the inferior mesenteric plexus.

The anus lies embedded in the soft tissue of the pelvis covered by an adventitia of loose connective tissue.

Multiple choice questions

1 Which of the following cell types is present in the small bowel and ascending colon but not in the descending colon?
   A Endocrine cells
   B Goblet cells
   C Paneth cells
   D Plasma cells
   E Eosinophils

2 Which of the following organs lacks lymphatic vessels in the lamina propria?
   A Esophagus
   B Stomach
   C Small bowel
   D Colon
   E All of the above

3 Which of the following choices correctly pairs the nerve plexi with their locations?
   A Meissner's plexus in lamina propria, Auerbach's plexus in submucosa
   B Meissner's plexus in submucosa, Auerbach's plexus in muscularis propria
   C Meissner's plexus in muscularis propria, Auerbach's plexus in muscularis mucosae
   D Meissner's plexus in muscularis mucosae, Auerbach's plexus in serosa
   E Meissner's plexus in serosa, Auerbach's plexus in lamina propria

4 Which of the following layers would be present in a mucosal biopsy?
   1) Lamina propria
   2) Muscularis propria
   3) Epithelium
   4) Serosa
   5) Submucosa
   6) Muscularis mucosae
   A 1, 3, 6
   B 2, 3, 5
   C 1, 2, 3, 5
   D 2, 4, 5
   E 3, 4, 5, 6

5 Which of the following cell types is not present in the body of the stomach?
   A Parietal cells
   B Chief cells
   C Enterochromaffin-like cells
   D Foveolar cells
   E G cells

References

1 Chandrasoma, P. (2003) Histopathology of the gastroesophageal junction: a study on 36 operation specimens. *The American Journal of Surgical Pathology*, **27**, 277–278.
2 Chandrasoma, P. (2003) Cardiac mucosal changes in a pediatric population. *The American Journal of Surgical Pathology*, **27**, 274–275; author reply 276–277.
3 Goldblum, J.R. (2000) Inflammation and intestinal metaplasia of the gastric cardia: Helicobacter pylori, gastroesophageal reflux disease, or both. *Digestive Diseases*, **18**, 14–19.
4 Kilgore, S.P., Ormsby, A.H., Gramlich, T.L. *et al*. (2000) The gastric cardia: fact or fiction? *The American Journal of Gastroenterology*, **95**, 921–924.
5 Owen, D.A. (1986) Normal histology of the stomach. *The American Journal of Surgical Pathology*, **10**, 48–61.
6 Pearse, A.G. and Riecken, E.O. (1967) Histology and cytochemistry of the cells of the small intestine, in relation to absorption. *British Medical Bulletin*, **23**, 217–222.
7 Levine, D.S. and Haggitt, R.C. (1989) Normal histology of the colon. *The American Journal of Surgical Pathology*, **13**, 966–984.
8 Tsang, P. and Rotterdam, H. (1999) Biopsy diagnosis of colitis: possibilities and pitfalls. *The American Journal of Surgical Pathology*, **23**, 423–430.

Answers

1 C
2 D
3 B
4 A
5 E

CHAPTER 2

Gastrointestinal hormones in the regulation of gut function in health and disease

John Del Valle

Department of Internal Medicine, Division of Gastroenterology, University of Michigan Medical Center, Ann Arbor, MI, USA

Introduction

GI hormones were first described by Bayliss and Starling [1] who identified a circulating substance derived from duodenal mucosa that caused pancreatic secretion when the duodenum was infused with acid. Numerous technical advances in the laboratory since then have contributed to our understanding of GI hormone biochemistry and physiology. It is now evident that GI hormones are short peptides. These peptides act as chemical messengers that facilitate communication between cells of the GI tract. They are involved in regulating numerous physiological gut functions, including intake, digestion, and absorption of nutrients; GI motility; gastroenteric pancreatic exocrine and endocrine secretion; and cellular growth and proliferation. In contrast to Bayliss and Starling who sought the chemical mediators responsible for physiological actions, we are now attempting to elucidate the biological function of identified substances and receptors [2, 3]. Our enhanced understanding of gut hormone biology has made it apparent that they may be involved in the pathophysiology of several clinical disorders and, additionally, may be useful as diagnostic and therapeutic tools.

Gut peptide classification and function

Structural analysis has uncovered striking similarities among several GI peptides. The basis of peptide homology is uncertain, but related peptides presumably have arisen through duplication of a common ancestral gene. Gut peptides with significant structural similarities have been grouped into hormone families (Table 2.1). After

Gastrointestinal Anatomy and Physiology: The Essentials, First Edition. Edited by John F. Reinus and Douglas Simon.
© 2014 John Wiley & Sons, Ltd. Published 2014 by John Wiley & Sons, Ltd.
www.wiley.com/go/reinus/gastro/anatomy

Table 2.1 GI hormone families.

Hormone family		Biological actions	Hormone family		Biological actions
Gastrin	Gastrin	↑ Acid secretion, ↑ Tissue proliferation	Pancreatic polypeptides	PP	↓ Pancreatic secretion
	CCK	↑ Pancreatic secretion, ↑ Gallbladder contraction		NPY	↑ Vasoconstriction, ↑ Food intake
	Secretin	↑ Pancreatic secretion		PYY	↓ Pancreatic secretion, ↓ Gastric secretion, ↓ Food intake
Secretin	Glucagon	↓ Intestinal motility	Tachykinin–bombesin	Substance K, P, Neurokinin	Contraction gut smooth muscle, Neurogenic inflammation
	VIP	↓ Smooth muscle contraction		GRP	↑ Gastrin release, ↑ Cell growth
	GLP-1	↑ Insulin secretion	SST	SS-14	↓ Acid secretion,
	GLP-2	↑ Cell growth		SS-34	↓ Pancreatic function, ↓ Cell growth
	GIP	↑ Insulin secretion	Motilin	Motilin	↑ GI motility
				Ghrelin	↑ Food intake

duplication, members of a gene family appear to have developed divergent structural and regulatory characteristics. GI hormones also may be classified according to cell of origin or biological action (neuropeptide, growth factor). Before describing the various GI hormone families, it is worth briefly reviewing several of the basic concepts related to hormone cells of origin, peptide synthesis, and receptor and postreceptor steps involved in hormone secretion.

Enteroendocrine cells

Gut hormones are synthesized and stored in specialized enteroendocrine cells (EECs) that are distributed throughout the GI tract. Together, these cells form the largest endocrine cell population in the body and produce the largest number of hormones of any endocrine organ [4]. One of the challenges in studying this system has been its diffuse and heterogeneous nature. Like endocrine cells found elsewhere in the body, EECs are highly specialized, stain with silver, and express specific neuroendocrine markers, such as chromogranin and neuron-specific enolase [5–10]. It was initially postulated that cells of the nervous system, endocrine organs, and enteroendocrine system with similar histologic character-istics are part of a diffuse neuroendocrine system that arises from the neural crest [11]. Subsequent molecular studies instead have shown that the EECs orig-inate from the endodermal epithelium [12]. Electron microscopy demonstrates that they are laden with secretory granules containing peptide hormones (Figure 2.1). Based on their morphology and peptide product, EECs have been categorized as being 1 of 16 types, each designated by a letter of the alphabet. It recently has been proposed, however, that cells should instead be named after the primary hormone or amine that they secrete and, when possible, their anatomic location [13].

Individual EECs are located in the epithelial layer of the GI tract and in pancreatic islets. They are characterized as being either open to the lumen and able to sample enteric contents or closed (no connection with the lumen). It is hypothesized that open-cell peptide secretion is triggered by luminal contents, such as nutrients and bacterial components. Pancreatic endocrine cells are closed. An additional important characteristic of many EECs is their ability to form long cytoplasmic processes that facilitate communication with adjacent targets, notably other cells. This unique trait was first recognized in gastric D cells, which were postulated to release their peptide product, Somatostatin, to inhibit G- and parietal cell activity [14]. Multiple additional cells subsequently have been found to form these processes, including ECL, K, I, and L cells. Recent elegant studies have found that the basal cytoplasmic processes of EECs increase in length from the proximal to the distal intestine [15]. These cellular appendages are filled with hormone vesicles and extend beneath the absorptive epithelium, resembling an axon that ends in a synapse-like bulb. The location and anatomy of these processes suggest that they monitor absorbed nutrients and convey electrochemical information to nerves and intestinal subepithelial myofibroblasts.

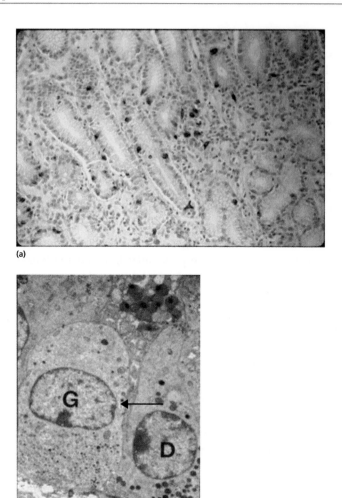

(a)

(b)

Figure 2.1 EEC of the GI tract. (a) Image of canine antral mucosa immunostained with a SST-specific antibody. Somatostatin cells are shown as the dark brown staining cells. This image depicts the small number and diffuse distribution of a typical EEC. (b) Electron micrograph of a gastrin and Somatostatin cell revealing the numerous secretory granules and the proximity of these cells to each other and to a capillary bed.

Synthesis and secretion

Synthesis and secretion of gut hormones involves a series of steps that occur within specialized cell compartments. The genes for the majority of GI peptides have been identified and fairly well characterized. As with proteins in general, peptide expression is controlled at the DNA level. Physiologic signals,

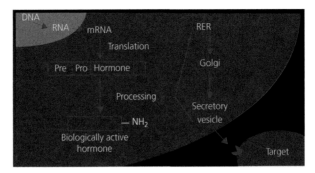

Figure 2.2 Diagram depicting the steps involved in the synthesis and processing of GI hormones. The process is initiated in the nucleus through gene transcription of the corresponding DNA into mRNA which in turn is translocated to the cytoplasm where it is translated into the corresponding precursor hormone, the preprohormone polypeptide chain. The precursor molecule is then processed through several steps in the rough endoplasmic reticulum (RER) and Golgi apparatus, resulting in the biologically active molecule which is stored in the secretory granule from which it is released to its target cell after a specific stimulus.

such as nutrient ingestion and duodenal acidification, will modify expression of genes for specific GI hormones. Negative feedback loops that shut off the action set in motion by a stimulus are built into these physiologic systems. GI hormones are synthesized through transcription of corresponding DNA into messenger RNA (mRNA) that, in turn, is translocated to the cytoplasm where it is translated into a precursor hormone, the preprohormone polypeptide chain (Figure 2.2). The preprohormone has a characteristic peptide sequence known as a signal peptide at its amino terminus that directs it to a ribosome of the rough endoplasmic reticulum (ER). Once bound to the ER, the signal peptide is cleaved, forming a prohormone that then is modified to form a biologically active peptide or hormone. The active molecule moves through the Golgi apparatus to the secretory granule where it is stored. The biochemical steps involved in making a prohormone an active molecule vary and can include many processes including amidation, glycosylation, phosphorylation, sulfation, and cleavage into peptides of differing lengths [17]. In fact, carboxyl-terminal amidation is important in over 50% of GI hormones and neurotransmitters. These posttranslational modifications determine the degree with which peptides bind to their receptors (see following text) and lead to a specific biological action [18]. There are also instances in which a single gene may be transcribed in several ways, leading to different hormone products. The classic example of this is production from a single gene of vasoactive intestinal polypeptide (VIP), neuromedin-A, and peptide histidine isoleucine (PHI) [19].

GI hormone-mediated action

As noted previously, GI hormones are important mediators of communication among key body regulatory systems. The forms of hormonal communication include the traditional endocrine route, a paracrine pathway (neurocrine, specialized paracrine), and an autocrine pathway (Figure 2.3) [2]. The endocrine route consists of delivery of a peptide hormone through the circulation to a distant target cell. In the paracrine pathway, GI peptides traverse the paracellular milieu to affect the function of an adjacent cell. The autocrine route involves hormonal influence on its cell of origin to regulate synthesis and secretion of additional peptide.

GI hormone receptors

GI hormones, often short hydrophilic peptides, bind to cell-surface receptors that span the hydrophobic cell membrane lipid bilayer and translate the binding action of ligands into downstream molecular intracellular events that lead to the physiological actions mediated by the target cells. There are three principal types of cell-surface receptors, each with different topography, that mediate GI hormone action: heptahelical G-protein-coupled receptors (GPCRs) (the most common receptor responsible for mediating GI hormone action) [20–22], ligand-gated channels that traverse the lipid bilayer multiple times and [23], and single transmembrane-type receptors that bind growth factors such as epidermal growth factor (EGF) [24].

The action of the vast majority of GI hormones is mediated through a member of the GPCR family [20–22, 25, 29]. GPCRs are the most common receptor type in the body; it is estimated that genes encoding the GPCR account for up to 5% of the genome in some mammals. GPCRs traverse the cell membrane seven times. They consist of an extracellular amino terminus,

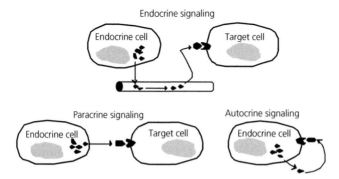

Figure 2.3 Pathways by which GI hormones mediate their actions. Once released, gut hormones can lead to subsequent target cell activation through either an endocrine (peptide reaches its target via the circulation), a paracrine (peptide traverses the paracellular environment to reach its target), or an autocrine (peptide acts upon its cell of origin).

lipophilic transmembrane domains, and an intracellular carboxyl terminus [20–26]. The ligands that bind to these receptors are diverse, ranging from photons to large viral particles. GPCRs are classified as being one of three general types based on their structural characteristics and those of their ligands. Class A (rhodopsin) receptors are small-molecule peptide ligands, class B receptors are large-polypeptide glucagon-like peptide-1 (GLP-1) ligands, and class C receptors are small-molecule glutamate ligands.

Postreceptor signaling

Upon binding its ligand, a receptor undergoes conformational changes that increase its affinity for a downstream G-protein effector that transduces the signal to a biological event (Figure 2.4). G-proteins consist of alpha, beta, and gamma subunits and are classified according to their alpha-subunit type. The alpha subunit contains the guanine-nucleotide binding site and has intrinsic GTPase activity [28–32]. G-protein activation follows a cyclic pattern. Upon G-protein binding, the beta and gamma (βγ) subunits dissociate from the alpha portion, which is bound to GDP under baseline conditions. GDP is then displaced by GTP. The GTP-bound alpha subunit activates a downstream target, for example, adenylate cyclase (AC), that in turn activates its downstream effector system. The GTPase activity of the alpha subunit cleaves a phosphate from GTP, converting it to GDP, which causes the alpha subunit to detach from the ligand receptor and bind to its corresponding βγ subunit, leaving it ready for the next cycle of activation. Activated alpha subunits interact with numerous effectors, including AC,

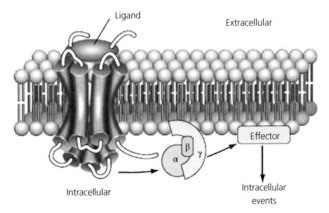

Figure 2.4 Receptor activation and postreceptor signaling. Diagram of a GPCR. As in the case of the gastrin receptor, GPCRs traverse the lipid bilayer of the cell membrane seven times. Upon ligand (gastrin) binding, the receptor undergoes conformational change which leads to binding of the corresponding G-protein, which, in turn, activates downstream effectors essential for the ultimate biological action (secretion, contraction, growth). From Reference [27].

phospholipases, guanylate cyclase, and ion channels. In addition, it is now clear that βγ subunits also can regulate numerous downstream effectors. A large number of mammalian genes for alpha subunits and βγ subunits set the stage for a multitude of potential combinations of these proteins, thus creating tremendous variety in downstream signaling possibilities. To prevent cell overstimulation, receptors are desensitized and internalized by events initiated within seconds of receptor activation. They are subsequently recycled to the cell surface, ready for the next round of cell activation.

GI hormone families

As noted previously, some GI hormones have been grouped into families on the basis of structural homology (Table 2.1).

Gastrin and cholecystokinin

Gastrin and cholecystokinin (CCK) are among the most thoroughly studied GI hormones [3, 17, 18]. They share a five-amino acid sequence at the carboxyl terminus that includes an amidated phenylalanine, which is important to the biological activity of this peptide family. In fact, carboxyl-terminal amidation turns out to be an important step in conferring biological activity on a large number of gut hormones [19]. Additional posttranslational modifications also are often important. For example, sulfation of the tyrosine located six amino acids away from the carboxyl-terminal phenylalanine is particularly important in making CCK biologically active (see following text).

Gastrin is synthesized primarily in antral G cells, but small quantities also are produced in endocrine cells of the small intestine and pancreas [33, 34]. G-cell activity is controlled by mediators that reach it through the circulation, the paracellular milieu, and neural pathways. In addition, it is a classic open cell, which implies that its activity may be affected by sampled luminal contents. Gastrin exists in several molecular forms, with the 17- and 34-amino acid variants being the most abundant (G17 and G34, respectively). Gastrin precursors, including the carboxy-terminal glycine-extended form and larger variants, also have been detected in tissue and the circulation [35]. The biological importance of gastrin-precursor forms has yet to be determined. It has been postulated that gastrin precursors may play a role in regulating cell proliferation in some malignancies, for example, colon cancer [36–40]. Gastrin activates its target through a GPCR similar to the receptor that binds CCK [41–44]. Originally referred to as CCK-A and CCK-B receptors, they have been renamed as CCK-1 and CCK-2, respectively. The genes and complimentary DNA (cDNA) sequences encoding the two receptors share 50% sequence homology. Ligand-binding studies demonstrate that the CCK-1 receptor has a one thousandfold greater affinity for CCK than for gastrin. Subsequent studies have documented that the CCK-2 receptor is the gastrin receptor found in the stomach [16].

Gastrin stimulates acid secretion and has a trophic effect on the gastric mucosa [45–47]. Acid secretion occurs through a dual mechanism: directly through stimulation of parietal cell-surface receptors and indirectly through stimulation of histamine release from ECL cells. Histamine, in turn, stimulates parietal cell acid secretion. Amino acids from peptides and proteins are the primary meal constituents that lead to gastrin release. This interaction is made possible by the G cell's open nature, which facilitates its exposure to luminal contents. Gastrin release also is stimulated by gastric distension. As in many other biological systems, a negative feedback loop stops acid production; low gastric pH turns off gastrin release through a hormonal pathway that involves the inhibitory GI peptide, Somatostatin (discussed in the following text). Gastrin's trophic effect plays a role in the physiologic maintenance of the gastric mucosa and has been theorized to play a pathophysiologic role in certain malignancies, including those of the colon, ovary, and stomach. Elevated serum gastrin levels can be due to a gastrin-producing tumor but more commonly result from natural or pharmacologic states of hypochlorhydria. Examples include pernicious anemia and atrophic gastritis associated with progression of chronic gastritis or more commonly from the use of acid-reducing agents, especially proton pump inhibitors (PPIs). The hypergastrinemia associated with atrophic gastritis has been thought to cause ECL hyperplasia and possible development of gastric carcinoid tumors (type I); although drug-induced hypergastrinemia has been found to cause gastric carcinoid tumors in rodents, this observation has not been made in humans, although reversible ECL hyperplasia has been associated with the use of PPIs in man.

CCK is secreted by small intestinal I cells in response to a meal [48]. It has been postulated that CCK release is in part mediated by a yet-to-be-isolated trypsin-sensitive CCK-releasing peptide (CCKrp). Trypsin-mediated degradation of CCKrp is postulated to serve as a built-in negative feedback mechanism for inhibiting further CCK release [49–51]. The main meal constituents responsible for stimulating CCK release are fat and protein. CCK acts upon a host of target organs through binding to the CCK-1 receptor. Targets include the gallbladder, pancreatic acinar cells, gastric smooth muscle, and peripheral nerves. CCK is a potent stimulant of gallbladder contraction and pancreatic secretion. It also plays a role in regulating gastric and intestinal motility. Finally, CCK appears to have a role in inducing satiety.

Secretin

The secretin family contains multiple hormones; those most relevant to GI function are highlighted in Table 2.1. Members of this family are relatively large peptides with substantial homology at the amino terminus. As noted earlier, secretin was discovered by Bayliss and Starling to stimulate pancreatic secretion [1]. It is released from small intestinal S cells in response to acidification of duodenal contents and is bound to a receptor on pancreatic acinar cells, leading to secretion of pancreatic fluid and bicarbonate, which are essential to neutralization of acid in chyme [52]. Secretin also acts on bile ductular epithelial, Brunner's gland, enteric smooth muscle, and EECs, producing other physiologic effects, including inhibition of gastric acid secretion (enterogastrone effect) and regulation of intestinal motility. Neutralization of duodenal pH stops secretin release. It has been postulated that acid-mediated stimulation of secretin release is caused by a protease-sensitive secretin-releasing factor [53]. Peptide hormones in the secretin family bind to a new class of GPCR [54, 55]. Structurally, these receptors are very similar to other GPCRs but have a unique long amino-terminal tail that contains six cysteine residues that are important for ligand binding and receptor activation.

VIP is a 28-amino acid peptide member of the secretin family that functions primarily as a neurotransmitter with numerous important actions in the GI tract and the central nervous system (CNS) [56]. VIP is found in and released from neurons. VIP-receptor binding activates the AC/cAMP pathway leading to a host of biological events including vasodilation, smooth muscle relaxation (particularly important in sphincter of Oddi and LES relaxation), and secretion of fluid and electrolytes from intestinal and biliary epithelial cells. VIP also may have immunomodulatory actions and regulatory effects on pancreatic and gastric secretion. Two VIP receptors (VIP1 and VIP2) of the secretin-family GPCR type have been cloned and characterized [57]. The receptors for VIP are distributed widely throughout the gut, consistent with its wide range of physiologic actions.

Glucagon is another well-known peptide member of the secretin family. It is a 29-amino acid peptide synthesized in and released from pancreatic alpha cells and L cells, which are found in the ileum and colon. Known as the insulin counterregulatory hormone, glucagon regulates glucose balance through stimulation of gluconeogenesis, lipolysis, and glycogenolysis. It is important to note that the gene for glucagon not only encodes preproglucagon but also encodes the precursor for GLP (GLP-1 and GLP-2) [58]. GLP-1 stimulates insulin secretion and enhances the stimulatory effect of glucose on insulin release from pancreatic islets. GLP-2 stimulates intestinal growth, enhancing mucosal mass. The glucagon receptor is also of the secretin-family GPCR type and is expressed in liver and skeletal muscle, where glucagon exerts its insulin counterregulatory effects.

Glucose-dependent insulinotropic peptide (GIP) was first thought to inhibit gastric acid secretion (thus initially named gastric inhibitory peptide) [59, 60]. Subsequently, it has become clear that the main biological action of this 42-amino acid peptide is to enhance glucose-dependent insulin secretion (incretin effect) [61]. GIP is synthesized in and secreted from proximal small intestinal mucosal K cells in the presence of luminal nutrients, specifically glucose and fat. It has significant structural homology with secretin and glucagon. GIP only increases insulin release in the presence of hyperglycemia. The GIP receptor is homologous with other receptors that bind this family of ligands and is expressed by the pancreatic beta cell and also by adipocytes, in which it increases triglyceride storage and fat accumulation.

Pancreatic polypeptide

Pancreatic polypeptide (PP), peptide YY (PYY), and neuropeptide Y (NPY) comprise the PP family [62, 63]. These three hormones have significant structural homology at the carboxyl terminus, which contains the biologically important and family-defining sequence of arginine–tyrosine amide. They bind to one of five homologous GPCRs and have relatively unique sites of origin and biological actions. PP is secreted from pancreatic endocrine cells and has numerous biological actions including the inhibition of pancreatic secretion, GI motility, and gallbladder contraction. NPY is a neurotransmitter that is abundant in the CNS and the peripheral nervous system. NPY has received much attention as an important appetite stimulant. PYY is expressed in EECs that are widely distributed throughout the gut but are most abundant in the ileum and colon. PYY was originally found to inhibit GI motility and chloride, gastric, and pancreatic secretion and was thus referred to as the ileal brake. Food is the main stimulant for PYY release, especially fat. Recently, PYY also has been shown to decrease appetite [64–66], a finding that has led to its consideration as a treatment for obesity.

Tachykinins and gastrin-releasing peptide (GRP)

The tachykinin family of GI hormones includes substance P and neurokinins A and B. These peptides are made by differential processing of the same preprotachykinin precursors and function primarily as neurotransmitters in both the CNS and peripheral nervous systems [67–69]. They each can bind to three different neurokinin receptors, NK-1, NK-2, or NK-3; however, substance P is the primary ligand for NK-1, neurokinin A the primary ligand for NK-2, and neurokinin B the primary ligand for NK-3. Substance P may be an important mediator of neurogenic inflammation in the gut. This hypothesis is supported by experimental models of bacterial colitis and the observation that substance P receptors are more abundant in the intestines of patients with inflammatory bowel disease (IBD) than in those of healthy controls [70, 71, 80, 81]. Several neuromedins also belong to the tachykinin hormone family. Four GPCRs (BB-1 through BB-4) bind these ligands.

Gastrin-releasing peptide (GRP) has substantial biochemical homology to the amphibian peptide, bombesin [72]. GRP is present in gastric neurons and stimulates gastrin secretion. It also may act as an excitatory neurotransmitter and a trophic factor.

Somatostatin

Somatostatin is found throughout the body, most notably in the gut [17, 18, 73]. It exists primarily in two molecular forms, SS-28 and, as the carboxyl-terminal end of SS-28, SS-14. A key disulfide bond between two cysteine residues makes

Somatostatin biologically active. Like many of the peptides discussed thus far, Somatostatin is expressed by and secreted from both GI neural and endocrine cells. In the gut, over 90% of Somatostatin is expressed in the mucosa. Well known for its inhibitory actions, Somatostatin can function via either endocrine, paracrine, or neurocrine pathways. Somatostatin cells in the stomach are unique in that they can have either an open (antrum) or a closed (body) configuration. In addition, some gastric Somatostatin endocrine cells have been found to have long neural-like processes abutting parietal or gastrin-producing cells. The later observation and the fact that Somatostatin cells in the antrum are "open" indicate that there is paracrine Somatostatin inhibition of gastrin release in response to acid secretion (negative feedback loop) [14]. The list of Somatostatin actions in the GI tract is extensive and includes the inhibition of gastric, pancreatic, bile, and intestinal secretion; reduction of splanchnic blood flow; inhibition of cell growth and proliferation; and inhibition of GI motility with, paradoxically, stimulation of the migrating motor complex (MMC). The later effect may be a dose-dependent phenomenon. Factors that stimulate Somatostatin release include low gastric pH, nutrients (fats and glucose), several GI hormones, and neural input. There are five Somatostatin GPCR subtypes [1–5], each with different tissue distribution and postreceptor coupling pathways. The broad inhibitory action of Somatostatin and the finding that a significant percentage of gut neuroendocrine tumors express Somatostatin receptors have led to the development of stable peptide Somatostatin analogues with both diagnostic and therapeutic applications [74].

Motilin

As its name implies, motilin is a key regulator of GI motility [75, 76]. Motilin is synthesized in and released from endocrine cells in the duodenal mucosa. It binds to specific GPCRs on GI smooth muscle to stimulate contraction and propulsive activity. Motilin is not stimulated by meal ingestion; it is released in a periodic or cyclic pattern that correlates with the initiation of MMC in the gut. Motilin receptors have been identified from the esophagus to the colon.

Ghrelin is a relatively new addition to the catalog of GI hormones [77, 78]. It was initially described as a ligand of the growth hormone secretagogue receptor. Ghrelin is a 28-amino acid peptide that plays a key role in regulating food intake and is the only known orexigenic (stimulant of food intake) gut hormone [79]. It has some structural homology with motilin, making it a member of this peptide's hormone family. Although ghrelin can stimulate gastric smooth muscle contraction, its main physiologic role is as an appetite stimulant. Within the GI tract, ghrelin is expressed in the stomach, pancreas, and intestine; the highest ghrelin concentrations are found in X/A-like cells of the oxyntic glands of the gastric fundus. Circulating ghrelin levels are highest in fasting and decrease after meals; animal studies have shown that central and peripheral ghrelin administration stimulates appetite. The peripheral effects of ghrelin are vagally mediated, while ghrelin acts centrally on NPY/agouti-related

Table 2.2 Clinical application of GI hormones.

GI hormone	Diagnostic study
Pentagastrin	Acid secretory studies
CCK	Biliary scanning
Secretin	Gastrin provocative testing Pancreatic function test
Glucagon	GI radiology Endoscopy
Somatostatin analogue	Radionuclide scanning

peptide (AgRP) neurons located in the arcuate nucleus of the hypothalamus. The gene that encodes ghrelin also encodes obestatin, a peptide initially thought to play a role in reducing food intake; however, the later action of obestatin has not been experimentally confirmed [79].

Conclusion

It has been evident since the turn of the last century that gut peptides are critical regulators of numerous GI functions. When the first endocrine neoplasms of the pancreas were described, it also became clear that excessive amounts of these same hormones play a role in the pathogenesis of disease, including the pathogenesis of obesity and inflammation [82, 83, 84]. Elucidation of gut hormone biology has made it obvious that they might also be used as diagnostic and therapeutic tools (Table 2.2).

Acknowledgments

The author would like to thank Karen Brown and Brian Minnich for their assistance in the preparation of this manuscript.

Multiple choice questions

1 Which of the following is the most common receptor type associated with GI hormone-mediated cell activation?
   A Intracellular transport receptor
   B G-protein-coupled receptor
   C Ligand-gated ion channel
   D Single transmembrane-type receptor

2 A 42-year-old male presents to your clinic with abdominal pain secondary to mild idiopathic chronic pancreatitis. You decide to manage the patient with pancreatic enzyme supplementation. Which of the following is the most likely mechanism for pancreatic enzyme replacement-mediated improvement of abdominal pain associated with chronic pancreatitis?

A Neutralization of duodenal secretion

B Breakdown of CCK-releasing peptide

C Breakdown of secretin-releasing peptide

D Induction of CCK-releasing peptide

E Induction of secretin-releasing peptide

References

1 Bayliss, W.M. and Starling, E.H. (1902 Sep) Mechanism of pancreatic secretion. *The Journal of Physiology*, **28** (5), 325–353.

2 Del Valle, J. and Yamada, T. (1990) The gut as an endocrine organ. *Annual Review of Medicine*, **41**, 447–455.

3 Del Valle, J. (1997) The stomach as an endocrine organ. *Digestion*, **58** (Suppl 1), 4–7.

4 Ahlman, H. and Nilsson, O. (2001) The gut as the largest endocrine organ in the body. *Annals of Oncology*, **12** (Suppl 2), S63–S68.

5 Sundler, F. (2004) GI tract, general anatomy (cells), in *Encyclopedia of Endocrine Diseases* (ed. L. Martini), Elsevier, Amsterdam, pp. 208–215.

6 Gunawardene, A.R., Corfe, B.M. and Staton, C.A. (2011) Classification and functions of enteroendocrine cells of the lower gastrointestinal tract. *International Journal of Experimental Pathology*, **92**, 219–231.

7 Modlin, I.M., Kidd, M., Pfragner, R. and Eick, G.N. (2006) Champaneria MC. The functional characterization of normal and neoplastic human enterochromaffin cells. *The Journal of Clinical Endocrinology and Metabolism*, **91**, 2340–2348.

8 Sakata, I. and Sakai, T. (2010) Ghrelin cells in the gastrointestinal tract. *International Journal of Peptides*, **2010**, 945056.

9 Stengel, A., Goebel, M., Yakubov, I. *et al.* (2009) Identification and characterization of nesfatin-1 immunoreactivity in endocrine cell types of the rat gastric oxyntic mucosa. *Endocrinology*, **150**, 232–238.

10 Cho, Y.M. and Kieffer, T.J. (2010) K-cells and glucose-dependent insulinotropic polypeptide in health and disease. *Vitamins and Hormones*, **84**, 111–150.

11 Modlin, I.M., Champaneria, M.C., Bornschein, J. and Kidd, M. (2006) Evolution of the diffuse enteroendocrine system–clear cells and cloudy origins. *Neuroendocrinology*, **84**, 69–82.

12 May, C.L. and Kaestner, K.H. (2010 Jul) Gut endocrine cell development. *Molecular and Cellular Endocrinology*, **323** (1), 70–75.

13 Helander, H.F. and Fändriks, L. (2012 Jan) The enteroendocrine "letter cells" – time for a new nomenclature? *Scandinavian Journal of Gastroenterology*, **47** (1), 3–12.

14 Larsson, L., Goltermann, N., de Magistris, L. *et al.* (1979 Sep) Somatostatin cell processes as pathways for paracrine secretion. *Science*, **205** (4413), 1393–1395.

15 Bohórquez, D.V. and Liddle, R.A. (2011 Oct) Axon-like basal processes in enteroendocrine cells: characteristics and potential targets. *Clinical and Translational Science*, **4** (5), 387–391.

16 Miller, L.J. (1990) Biochemical characterization of receptors for the cholecystokinin family of hormones, in *Gastrointestinal Endocrinology: Receptors and Post-Receptor Mechanisms* (ed. J.C. Thompson), Academic Press, New York, p. 81.

17 Rehfeld, J.F. (1998 Apr) Processing of precursors of gastroenteropancreatic hormones: diagnostic significance. *Journal of Molecular Medicine (Berl)*, **76** (5), 338–345.

18 Itoh, K.O., Obata, K., Yanaihara, N. and Okamoto, H. (1983 Aug) Human preprovasoactive intestinal polypeptide contains a novel PHI-27-like peptide, PHM-27. *Nature*, **304** (5926), 547–549.

19 Dohlman, H.G., Caron, M.G. and Lefkowitz, R.J. (1987 May) A family of receptors coupled to guanine nucleotide regulatory proteins. *Biochemistry*, **26** (10), 2657–2664.

20 Ji, T.H., Grossmann, M. and Ji, I. (1998 Jul) G protein-coupled receptors. *Journal of Molecular Medicine*, **273** (28), 17299–17302.

21 Lefkowitz, R.J. (2000 Jul) The superfamily of heptahelical receptors. *Nature Cell Biology*, **2** (7), E133–E136.

22 Luetje, C.W., Patrick, J. and Seguela, P. (1990 Jul) Nicotine receptors in the mammalian brain. *Journal of Federation of American Societies for Experimental Biology*, **4** (10), 2753–2760.

23 Brown, K.D. (1995 Oct) The epidermal growth factor/transforming growth factor-alpha family and their receptors. *European Journal of Gastroenterology & Hepatology*, **7** (10), 914–922.

24 McCudden, C.R., Hains, M.D., Kimple, R.J. *et al.* (2005) G-protein signaling: back to the future. *Cellular and Molecular Life Sciences*, **62**, 551–577.

25 Tuteje, N. (2009) Signaling through G protein coupled receptors. *Plant Signaling & Behavior*, **4** (10), 942–994.

26 Gilman, A.G. (1987) G proteins: transducers of receptor-generated signals. *Annual Review of Medicine*, **56**, 615–649.

27 Liddle, R.A. (2010) Gastrointestinal hormones and neurotransmitters, in *Sleisenger and Fordtran's Gastrointestinal and Liver Disease*, 9th edn (ed. M. Feldman), Saunders, Philadelphia, pp. 3–19.

28 Birnbaumer, L. (1990) G proteins in signal transduction. *Annual Review of Pharmacology and Toxicology*, **30**, 675–705.

29 Neer, E.J. and Clapham, D.E. (1988 May) Roles of G protein subunits in transmembrane signalling. *Nature*, **333** (6169), 129–134.

30 Patel, T.B. (2004 Sep) Single transmembrane spanning heterotrimeric G protein–coupled receptors and their signaling cascades. *Pharmacological Reviews*, **56** (3), 371–385.

31 Pierce, K.L., Premont, R.T. and Lefkowitz, R.J. (2002 Sep) Seven-transmembrane receptors. *Nature Reviews Molecular Cell Biology*, **3** (9), 639–650.

32 Walsh, J.H. (1987) Gastrointestinal hormones, in *Physiology of the Gastrointestinal Tract* (ed. L.R. Johnson), Raven Press, New York, p. 181.

33 Brand, S.J. and Fuller, P.J. (1988 Apr) Differential gastrin gene expression in rat gastrointestinal tract and pancreas during neonatal development. *Journal of Molecular Medicine*, **263** (11), 5341–5347.

34 Del Valle, J., Sugano, K. and Yamada, T. (1989 Nov) Glycine-extended processing intermediates of gastrin and cholecystokinin in human plasma. *Gastroenterology*, **97** (5), 1159–1163.

35 Kochman, M.L., Del Valle, J., Dickinson, C.J. and Boland, C.R. (1992) Post-translational processing of gastrin in neoplastic colonic tissues. *Biochemical and Biophysical Research Communications*, **189**, 1165–1169.

36 van Solinge, W.W., Nielsen, F.C., Friis-Hansen, L. *et al.* (1993 Apr) Expression but incomplete maturation of progastrin in colorectal carcinomas. *Gastroenterology*, **104** (4), 1099–1107.

37 Dickinson, C.J. (1995 Oct) Relationship of gastrin processing to colon cancer. *Gastroenterology*, **109** (4), 1384–1388.

38 Wang, T.C., Koh, T.J., Varro, A. *et al.* (1996 Oct) Processing and proliferative effects of human progastrin in transgenic mice. *Journal of Clinical Investigation*, **98** (8), 1918–1929.

39 Dockray, G.J. (2000 Dec) Gastrin, growth, and colon neoplasia. *Gut*, **47** (6), 747–748.

40 Aly, A., Shulkes, A. and Baldwin, G.S. (2004 Jul) Gastrins, cholecystokinins and GI cancer. *Biochimica et Biophysica Acta*, **1704** (1), 1–10.

41 Soll, A.H., Amirian, D.A., Thomas, L.P. *et al.* (1984 May) Gastrin receptors on isolated canine parietal cells. *Journal of Clinical Investigation*, **73** (5), 1434–1447.

42 Kopin, A.S., Lee, Y.M., McBride, E.W. *et al.* (1992 Apr) Expression cloning and characterization of the canine parietal cell gastrin receptor. *Proceedings of the National Academy of Sciences of the United States of America*, **89** (8), 3605–3609.

43 Wank, S.A. (1995 Nov) Cholecystokinin receptors. *American Journal of Physiology*, **269** (5 Pt 1), G628–G646.

44 Soll, A. (1978 Feb) The interaction of histamine with gastrin and carbamylcholine on oxygen uptake by isolated mammal parietal cells. *Journal of Clinical Investigation*, **61** (2), 381–389.

45 Willems, G., Vansteenkiste, Y. and Limbosch, J.M. (1972 Apr) Stimulating effect of gastric on cell proliferation kinetics in canine fundic mucosa. *Gastroenterology*, **62** (4), 583–589.

46 Rehfeld, J.F. (1998 Oct) The new biology of GI hormones. *Physiological Reviews*, **78** (4), 1087–1108.

47 Liddle, R.A. (1994) Cholecystokinin, in *Gut Peptides: Biochemistry and Physiology* (eds J.H. Walsh and G.J. Dockray), Raven Press, New York p. 175.

48 Iwai, K., Fukuoka, S., Fushiki, T. *et al.* (1987 Jul) Purification and sequencing of a trypsin-sensitive cholecystokinin-releasing peptide from rat pancreatic juice. Its homology with pancreatic secretory trypsin inhibitor. *Journal of Molecular Medicine*, **262** (19), 8956–8959.

49 Herzig, K.H., Schon, I., Tatemoto, K., *et al.* (1996 Jul) Diazepam binding inhibitor is a potent cholecystokinin-releasing peptide in the intestine. *Proceedings of the National Academy of Sciences of the United States of America*, **93** (15), 7927–7932.

50 Li, Y., Hao, Y. and Owyang, C. (2000 Feb) Diazepam-binding inhibitor mediates feedback regulation of pancreatic secretion and postprandial release of cholecystokinin. *Journal of Clinical Investigation*, **105** (3), 351–359.

51 Leiter, A.B., Chey, W.Y. and Kopin, A.S. (1994) Secretin, in *Gut Peptides: Biochemistry and Physiology* (eds J.H. Walsh and G.J. Dockray), Raven Press, New York, p. 144.

52 Li, P., Lee, K.Y., Chang, T.M. and Chey, W.Y. (1990 Nov) Mechanism of acid-induced release of secretin in rats. Presence of a secretin-releasing peptide. *Journal of Clinical Investigation*, **86** (5), 1474–1479.

53 Ishihara, T., Nakamura, S., Kaziro, Y. *et al.* (1991 July) Molecular cloning and expression of a cDNA encoding the secretin receptor. *The EMBO Journal*, **10** (7), 1635–1641.

54 Ishihara, T., Shigemoto, R., Mori, K. *et al.* (1992 Apr) Functional expression and tissue distribution of a novel receptor for vasoactive intestinal tissue distribution of a novel receptor for vasoactive intestinal polypeptide. *Neuron*, **8** (4), 811–819.

55 Dockray, G.J. (1994) Vasoactive intestinal polypeptide and related peptides, in *Gut Peptides: Biochemistry and Physiology* (eds J.H. Walsh and G.J. Dockray), Raven Press, New York, p. 447.

56 Usdin, T.B., Bonner, T.I. and Mezey, E. (1994 Dec) Two receptors for vasoactive intestinal polypeptide with similar specificity and complementary distributions. *Endocrinology*, **135** (6), 2662–2680.

57 Drucker, D.J. (1998 Feb) Glucagon-like peptides. *Diabetes*, **47** (2), 159–169.

58 Moody, A.J., Thim, L. and Valverde, I. (1984 Jul) The isolation and sequencing of human gastric inhibitory polypeptide (GIP). *FEBS Letters*, **172** (2), 142–148.

59 Usdin, T.B., Mezey, E., Button, D.C. *et al.* (1993 Dec) Gastric inhibitory polypeptide receptor, a member of the secretin-vasoactive intestinal peptide receptor family, is widely distributed in peripheral organs and the brain. *Endocrinology*, **133** (6), 2861–2870.

60 Pederson, R.A. (1994) Gastric inhibitory polypeptide, in *Gut Peptides: Biochemistry and Physiology* (eds J.H. Walsh and G.J. Dockray), Raven Press, New York, p. 217.

61 Hazelwood, R.L. (1993 Jan) The pancreatic polypeptide (PP-fold) family: gastrointestinal, vascular, and feeding behavioral implications. *Proceedings of the Society for Experimental Biology and Medicine*, **202** (1), 44–63.

62 Mannon, P. and Taylor, I.L. (1994) The pancreatic polypeptide family, in *Gut Peptides: Biochemistry and Physiology* (eds J.H. Walsh and G.J. Dockray), Raven Press, New York, p. 341.

63 Stanley, S., Wynne, K. and Bloom, S. (2004 May) Gastrointestinal satiety signals III. Glucagon-like peptide 1, oxyntomodulin, peptide YY, and pancreatic polypeptide. *American Journal of Physiology: Gastrointestinal and Liver Physiology*, **286** (5), G693–G697.

64 Suzuki, K., Simpson, K.A., Minnion, J.S. *et al.* (2010) The role of gut hormones and the hypothalamus in appetite regulation. *Endocrine Journal*, **57** (5), 359–372.

65 Batterham, R.L., Cohen, M.A., Ellis, S.M. *et al.* (2003 Sep) Inhibition of food intake in obese subjects by peptide YY3–36. *The New England Journal of Medicine*, **349** (10), 941–948.

66 Improta, G. and Broccardo, M. (2006 Aug) Tachykinins: role in human gastrointestinal tract physiology and pathology. *Current Drug Targets*, **7** (8), 1021–1029.

67 Satake, H. and Kawada, T. (2006 Aug) Overview of the primary structure, tissue-distribution, and functions of tachykinins and their receptors. *Current Drug Targets*, **7** (8), 963–974.

68 Pennefather, J.N., Lecci, A., Candenas, M.L. *et al.* (2004 Feb) Tachykinins and tachykinin receptors: a growing family. *Life Sciences*, **74** (12), 1445–1463.

69 Mantyh, C.R., Pappas, T.N., Lapp, J.A. *et al.* (1996 Nov) Substance P activation of enteric neurons in response to intraluminal Clostridium difficile toxin A in the rat ileum. *Gastroenterology*, **111** (5), 1272–1280.

70 Mantyh, P.W., Mantyh, C.R., Gates, T. *et al.* (1988 Jun) Receptor binding sites for substance P and substance K in the canine gastrointestinal tract and their possible role in inflammatory bowel disease. *Neuroscience*, **25** (3), 817–837.

71 Lebacq-Verheyden, A.M., Trepel, J., Sausville, E.A. and Battey, J.F. (1991) Bombesin and gastrin-releasing peptide: neuropeptides, secretagogues, and growth factors, in *Peptide Growth Factors and Their Receptors* (eds M.B. Sporn and A.B. Roberts), Springer-Verlag, Heidelberg, p. 71.

72 Chiba, T. and Yamada, T. (1994) Gut somatostatin, in *Gut Peptides: Biochemistry and Physiology* (eds J.H. Walsh and G.J. Dockray), Raven Press, New York, p. 123.

73 Del Valle, J. (1993) Application of somatostatin and its analogue octreotide in the therapy of gastrointestinal disorders, in *Gastrointestinal Pharmacotherapy* (ed. M.M. Wolfe), W.B. Saunders, Philadelphia, p. 275.

74 Depoortere, I. (2001) Motilin and motilin receptors: characterization and functional significance. *Verhandelingen – Koninklijke Academie voor Geneeskunde van België*, **63** (6), 511–529.

75 Peeters, T.L. and Depoortere, I. (1994 Dec) Motilin receptor: a model for development of prokinetics. *Digestive Diseases and Sciences*, **39** (Suppl 12), 76S–78S.

76 Kojima, M., Hosoda, H., Date, Y. *et al.* (1999 Dec) Ghrelin is a growth-hormone-releasing acylated peptide from stomach. *Nature*, **402** (6762), 656–660.

77 Kojima, M. and Kangawa, K. (2005 Apr) Ghrelin: structure and function. *Physiological Reviews*, **85** (2), 495–522.

78 Karra, E. and Batterham, R.L. (2010 Mar) The role of gut hormones in the regulation of body weight and energy homeostasis. *Molecular and Cellular Endocrinology*, **316** (2), 120–128.

79 Del Valle, J. (2009) Zollinger-Ellison Syndrome, in *Textbook of Gastroenterology*, 5th edn (ed. T. Yamada), Lippincott, Philadelphia, pp. 982–1004.

80 Mantyh, P.W., Mantyh, C.R., Gates, T. *et al.* (1988) Receptor binding sites for substance P and substance K in the canine gastrointestinal tract and their possible role in inflammatory bowel disease. *NeuroScience*, **25**, 817–837.

81 Genton, L. and Kudsk, K.A. (2003) Interactions between the enteric nervous system and the immune system: role of neuropeptides and nutrition. *The American Journal of Surgery*, **186**, 253–258.

82 Field, A.E., Coakley, E.H., Must, A. *et al.* (2001) Impact of overweight on the risk of developing common chronic diseases during a 10-year period. *Archives of Internal Medicine*, **161**, 1581–1586.

83 Must, A., Spadano, J., Coakley, E.H. *et al.* (1999) The disease burden associated with overweight and obesity. *The Journal of the American Medical Association*, **282**, 1523–1529.

84 Cummings, D.E. and Overduin, J. (2007 Jan) Gastrointestinal regulation of food intake. *Journal of Clinical Investigation*, **117** (1), 13–23.

Answers

1 B

2 B. Chronic pancreatitis is theorized to lead to a relative increase of CCK releasing peptide (CCK rp) due to the deficiency in trypsin, which is the natural mediator of CCK rp breakdown. The increased CCK rp, then leads to a tonic increase in CCK release, which is believed to increase pancreatic enzyme secretion which in turn leads to worsening pain. Providing the pancreatic enzymes restores the negative feedback loop by destroying the trypsin sensitive CCK rp and therefore decreasing further CCK release.

CHAPTER 3

Gastrointestinal motility

Ikuo Hirano & Darren Brenner

Division of Gastroenterology, Northwestern University Feinberg School of Medicine, Chicago, IL, USA

Introduction

Motility is essential to GI function. Motility is involved in swallowing, gastric mechanical digestion, gastric emptying, intestinal absorption of nutrients and water, and defecation. This chapter reviews the physiology of gastrointestinal (GI) motility.

Enteric nervous system

The enteric nervous system (ENS), often referred to as the second brain, is comprised of over 100 million neurons that provide local neural control of many GI functions. The ENS consists of two plexi: Meissner's (submucous) plexus between the muscularis mucosa and the circular muscle layer of the gut and the myenteric plexus between the circular and longitudinal muscle layers of the gut. The ENS contains over 20 neurotransmitters that affect motility, secretion, gut microcirculation, and immunologic function (Table 3.1). Many prokinetic and inhibitory agents used in gastrointestinal motility disorders have actions that involve the neurotransmitters of the ENS (Table 3.2, 3.3).

The ENS is connected to the central nervous system (CNS) by parasympathetic and sympathetic nerves (Figure 3.1). Parasympathetic fibers reach the gut through the vagus nerve and sacral outflow tracts. Although the vagus nerve has connections with the GI organs from the pharynx to the proximal colon, its principal motility effects are on the esophagus and stomach. Projections of the vagus nerve directly innervate the pharynx and striated muscle of the esophagus. Vagal innervation of GI smooth muscle is indirect, via the ENS. The vagus nerve also is involved in secretomotor activity of the stomach and gallbladder. Preganglionic neurons in the S1–S5 region of the spinal cord (sacral outflow) innervate the distal colon and anal sphincter.

Gastrointestinal Anatomy and Physiology: The Essentials, First Edition. Edited by John F. Reinus and Douglas Simon.
© 2014 John Wiley & Sons, Ltd. Published 2014 by John Wiley & Sons, Ltd.
www.wiley.com/go/reinus/gastro/anatomy

Table 3.1 Putative neurotransmitters of the ENS.

Amines	Peptides
ACh	Calcitonin gene-related peptide
Norepinephrine	cholecystokinin
Serotonin (5-hydroxytryptamine)	Galanin
Amino acids	gastrin-releasing peptide
Glutamate	Neuromedin U
Glycine	neuropeptide Y
Gamma aminobutyric acid	Neurotensin
Purines	Opioids
ATP	peptide YY
Adenosine	Pituitary adenylate cyclase-activating polypeptide
Gases	SST
NO	Substance P
	Thyrotropin-releasing hormone
	Vasoactive intestinal contractor
	VIP

Table 3.2 Prokinetic therapies used in GI motility disorders.

Agent	Mechanism of action	Site of action
Metoclopramide (Reglan®)	Dopamine receptor (D2) antagonist	ENS CNS
Cisapride (Propulsid®)	Stimulates ACh release, 5HT4 agonist 5HT3 antagonist	ENS
Erythromycin	Motilin receptor agonist	ENS (ACh neurons) Smooth muscle
Domperidone	Dopamine receptor (D2) antagonist	ENS
Octreotide	Stimulates MMC Decrease antral motility	? ENS ? Hormone
Tegaserod (Zelnorm®)	5HT4 partial agonist	ENS (ACh neurons)
Neostigmine	Acetylcholinesterase inhibitor	ENS (ACh neurons)

Sympathetic neural control of gut function originates in preganglionic cholinergic neurons in the spinal cord that synapse with postganglionic noradrenergic neurons in the celiac, superior mesenteric, inferior mesenteric, and pelvic ganglia. Sympathetic efferent stimulation generally inhibits GI motor and secretory function by decreasing release of acetylcholine (ACh) from enteric neurons. These

Table 3.3 Inhibitory pharmacologic therapies used in GI motility disorders.

Agent	Mechanism of action	Site of action
Nitrates (sublingual, PO, topical)	NO donor	Smooth muscle
Sildenafil, tadalafil, vardenafil	Selective inhibition cGMP phosphodiesterase 5; increase cGMP (second messenger for NO)	Smooth muscle
Nifedipine, amlodipine, diltiazem	Calcium channel antagonist	Smooth muscle
Botulinum toxin	Inhibit exocytosis of ACh from nerve endings	ENS
Dicyclomine, atropine, methscopolamine, hyoscyamine	ACh receptor antagonist	ENS
Alosetron	5HT3 receptor antagonist	ENS

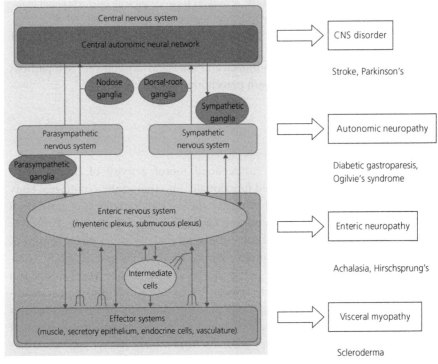

Figure 3.1 Schematic depiction of the neurologic control of GI motility. The central, autonomic, and enteric nervous systems work in concert on the smooth muscle effector system of the GI tract. Disorders at each level of neurologic control or at the visceral smooth muscle end organ level may result in motility disorders. Specific examples of disorders are listed to the right side of the schematic. Adapted from Reference [1].

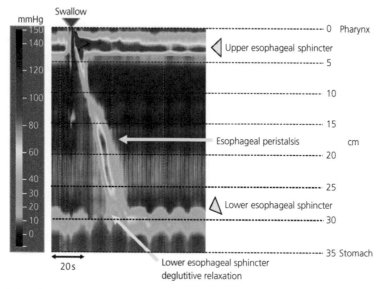

Figure 3.2 Isobaric color contour plot of normal esophageal manometry. Color denotes the amplitude of esophageal contractile activity. A swallow is associated with brief relaxation of the upper esophageal sphincter followed by sequential contractions of the esophageal body comprising primary peristalsis. Relaxation of the LES corresponds with the onset of swallowing.

effects are most prominent in the stomach and small and large bowels. Sympathetic afferent nerves mediate visceral pain perception (nociception).

Esophageal motility

Esophageal motility is the best understood motor activity of the GI tract. Esophageal motility can be divided functionally into that of the esophageal body and that of the lower esophageal sphincter (LES). Body motility is characterized by sequential (peristaltic) contractions of circular muscle (Figure 3.2). Peristalsis in the smooth muscle segment of the esophageal body is under direct control of the ENS. Excitatory cholinergic enteric neurons and inhibitory nitric oxide (NO)-generating neurons coordinate peristaltic waves of muscle contraction and relaxation: cholinergic neurons are responsible for the amplitude of muscle contraction, and NO neurons are responsible for the inhibitory phase that precedes contraction. This inhibitory phase lengthens as it moves down the esophagus, a phenomenon known as the latency gradient. Inhibition of NO synthase abolishes the latency gradient, resulting in simultaneous muscle contractions. This motility pattern mimics that seen in patients with achalasia and diffuse esophageal spasm.

The second functional portion of the esophagus, the LES, is ordinarily closed, forming the major barrier to reflux of gastric contents. The LES opens in response to a variety of stimuli, including swallowing (primary peristalsis) (Figure 3.2), esophageal distension (secondary peristalsis), and gastric distension (as occurs

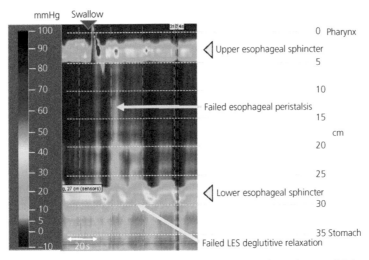

Figure 3.3 Isobaric color contour plot of achalasia. Complete esophageal aperistalsis is event with failure of deglutitive relaxation of the LES.

in transient LES relaxation). LES resting pressure is maintained by myogenic and neurogenic inputs, whereas LES relaxation occurs in response to neurogenic input alone. The intrinsic ability of LES smooth muscle to remain contracted in the absence of external neural or hormonal influences is referred to as myogenic tone. Esophageal body smooth muscle, in contrast, generally does not have myogenic tone. The myenteric plexus is the source of LES neurogenic input. The myenteric plexus contains both excitatory and inhibitory motor neurons. Excitatory neurons release neurotransmitters such as ACh that stimulate the smooth muscle contraction responsible for LES resting tone. Inhibitory neurons release neurotransmitters such as NO and VIP that cause LES relaxation. Experimental NO inhibition results in the elevation of basal LES pressure and loss of swallow-induced relaxation. This manometric pattern mimics that seen in patients with achalasia (Figure 3.3). Studies have demonstrated the absence of NO neurons in the myenteric plexi of patients with achalasia [1].

Gastric motility

The stomach can be divided into two functional areas: the body and the fundus. Both actively relax during a meal. This accommodation reflex is a vagally mediated event that allows ingested food to accumulate in the fundus where it can be acted on by gastric acid and pepsin. The gastric fundus generates tonic and short-duration phasic contractions that gradually transfer ingested food to the antrum. These contractions promote gastric emptying by creating a pressure gradient between the stomach and the duodenum. The gastric antrum and pylorus function in concert to mechanically digest food. The antrum generates high-amplitude phasic contractions that forcefully propel food against a closed pylorus.

In doing so, the antrum triturates, or grinds, solid material to particles 1.0–2.0 mm in diameter. The pylorus acts as a sieve by preventing the passage of larger particles. Small particle size maximizes the ratio of surface area to volume, optimizing food exposure to small bowel digestive enzymes. Following completion of this process, larger indigestible gastric contents are emptied by the migrating motor complex (MMC). The MMC has three phases: a period of quiescence (phase 1), a period of intermittent pressure activity (phase 2), and a period of high-amplitude contractile waves that, in the case of the stomach, propel residual gastric contents through an open pylorus into the duodenum (phase 3). This sequence of events occurs approximately every 60–90 min during the interdigestive period.

Slow waves of spontaneous rhythmic electrical depolarization control the frequency of gastric smooth muscle contraction. They originate in the interstitial cells of Cajal (ICCs) located in the pacemaker region of the stomach on the greater curvature between the fundus and the proximal body. These cells are intercalated between nerve endings and smooth muscle cells and have spontaneous rhythmic electrical activity known as pacesetter potentials that propagate circumferentially with a frequency of three cycles per minute. ICCs are found in the GI tract from the stomach to the colon.

The nature of ingested material determines the kinetics of gastric emptying. Liquids have a half-life in the stomach of approximately 20–30 min and solids a half-life of approximately 60–90 min. The slower emptying of solids is due to the time required for mechanical digestion. The actual emptying time of food also depends on its calorie and fat content. In the postprandial period, the MMC is replaced by irregular contractions of variable frequency and amplitude. The duration of this motility pattern is directly proportional to the calorie content of the meal. Feedback inhibition of gastric muscle contraction initiated by chemo-receptors in the duodenum delays gastric emptying of fat, glucose, and hyper-tonic fluids. Large indigestible solids, such as timed-release medication capsules and fibrous foods, are emptied from the stomach during the third phase of the MMC. The MMC is inhibited for more than 2 h after the fed state.

Receptive relaxation and accommodation in the gastric fundus and body are mediated by the vagus nerve. The loss of the accommodation reflex in patients who have undergone vagotomy is responsible for accelerated liquid emptying. Vagotomy also interferes with antral contractile activity, which delays mechanical digestion and therefore emptying of solids. This is the reason why patients undergoing vagotomy require pyloroplasty [2].

Small bowel motility

Small intestinal muscle contractions mix digested food with pancreatic enzymes, bile, and intestinal secretions and propel it across the intestinal mucosa where it can be further digested and absorbed. The small intestine has two distinct motility

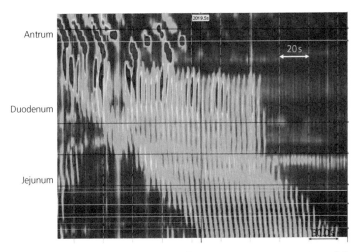

Figure 3.4 Isobaric color contour plot of phase 3 of the MMC. Phasic contractions of the gastric antrum occur at a slower frequency than clustered contractions of the duodenum and jejunum.

patterns: a fed pattern and a fasting pattern. The fed pattern is characterized by segmentation: nonpropagated focal contractions of intestine that occur simultaneously at multiple locations in the intestine. This pattern typically lasts 4–6 h following a meal and is replaced by the fasting pattern. The fasting pattern of small bowel motility is dominated by the MMC, as previously described (Figure 3.4). In the small bowel, phase 3 serves to sweep debris and bacteria out of the intestine.

The local peristaltic reflex is one of the better understood small bowel motor patterns. In this reflex, a food bolus in the gut lumen stimulates mucosal afferent nerves. A series of interneurons activate motor neurons containing excitatory transmitters such as ACh and substance P proximal to the bolus and motor neurons containing inhibitory transmitters such as NO and VIP distal to the bolus. The net result is aboral propagation of contraction above and relaxation below the bolus.

Chemoreceptors throughout the small bowel help to regulate gastric emptying and control the rate of nutrient delivery to the small bowel. An example of this activity is the "ileal brake," whereby ileal fat delays gastric emptying. Proposed mediators of the ileal brake include peptide YY, enteroglucagon, and neurotensin [2].

Colonic motility

Enteric contents are continually delivered to the colon in the fed and fasting states. The colon stores feces until such time as it can be evacuated conveniently. Fecal storage facilitates maximal absorption of water, electrolytes, short-chain fatty acids, and bacterial metabolites. Colonic motility, like gastric and small bowel motility, is under the involuntary control of the ENS.

Motor activity in the ascending colon is characterized by ring contractions that migrate proximally. This reverse peristalsis promotes temporary fecal retention. The contents of the transverse and descending colons are generally pushed caudally by mass movement: lumen-obliterating intermittent contractions of colonic circular muscle that propel feces short distances. As a result of mass movement, feces gradually moves from the right colon where it was initially stored to the sigmoid colon and rectum. Mass movement is a motility pattern that is not regulated by intrinsic slow-wave activity. Instead, it has been proposed that mass movements are under autonomic control, as they can be initiated by stimulation of parasympathetic sacral outflow tracts.

The gastrocolic reflex and the giant peristaltic contraction are propulsive contractile patterns unique to the colon. The gastrocolic reflex increases colonic motility within 30 min of a meal. It is stimulated by food in the duodenum and appears to be a neurally mediated response that involves cholecystokinin release. The giant peristaltic contraction is a peristaltic reflex characterized by high-amplitude and long-duration contractions. This reflex can be induced by cholera toxin and is found in some patients with irritable bowel syndrome. Its electrical correlate is known as the migrating action potential complex [2].

Anorectal motility

The anorectum has both smooth (internal anal sphincter) and skeletal (external anal sphincter and puborectalis) muscle components that maintain fecal continence and allow voluntary control of defecation. The puborectalis originates from the posterior aspect of the pubic bone and forms a sling around the rectum. It is tonically contracted at rest, creating an acute angle between the levator ani and external anal sphincter muscles. This sharp angle assists in maintaining normal continence. The external anal sphincter muscles are innervated by the pudendal nerve with fibers originating from S2 to S4. They are responsible for 15–20% of resting sphincter tone, but the external sphincter muscles are 100% responsible for maintaining fecal continence when a conscious decision is made to avoid defecation. Phasic contractions of the puborectalis and external anal sphincter muscles also contribute to the preservation of fecal continence. These contractions are important during periods of increased intra-abdominal pressure, for example, during coughing, laughing, sneezing, changes in posture, and lifting of heavy objects. The internal anal sphincters are smooth muscles innervated by sympathetic and parasympathetic fibers from the sacral plexus. Input from both types of fibers is inhibitory and keeps the sphincter in a constant state of contraction at rest. The internal anal sphincter is responsible for 80–85% of resting anal sphincter tone and is the primary deterrent to involuntary defecation.

Defecation is a complex process characterized by coordination of the abdominal- and pelvic-floor musculature and the internal and external anal

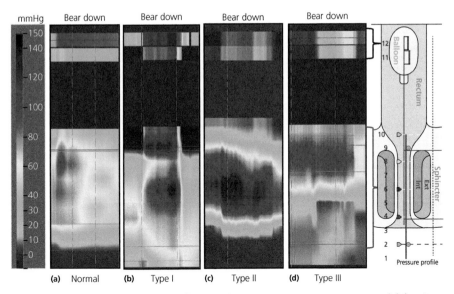

Figure 3.5 Isobaric color contour plots of anorectal manometric responses to attempted defecation.
(a) Normal pattern: There is an appropriate increase in intrarectal pressure (black parenthesis;
>45 mm Hg) with reflexive relaxation of the anal sphincters (red parenthesis). (b) Type I
dyssynergia: There is an appropriate increase in intrarectal pressure but paradoxical contraction of
the anal sphincters. (c) Type II dyssynergia: There is an insufficient increase in intrarectal pressure
with paradoxical contraction of the anal sphincters. This is also known as inadequate defecatory
propulsion. (d) Type III dyssynergia: There is an appropriate increase in intrarectal pressure with
a lack of anal sphincter relaxation.

sphincters. Normal defecation begins with a Valsalva maneuver that increases
intra-abdominal pressure. The pressure is transmitted to the pelvis, resulting in
relaxation of the puborectalis muscle, widening of the anorectal angle, and
relaxation of the internal anal sphincters. The pelvic floor descends, and the
external anal sphincter is voluntarily relaxed. If the pressure in the rectum is
greater than the pressures across the anal sphincters (i.e., a positive pressure
gradient), stool is evacuated. Failure of any of these steps can lead to diffi-
culties with defecation. Dyssynergic defecation, the most common evacuation
disorder, also is known as anismus, obstructive defecation, and pelvic-floor
dyssynergia. It is characterized by poor coordination of abdominal- and pelvic-
floor musculature during attempted defecation and has been classified into
three distinct subtypes: type I, generation of appropriate intrarectal pressure
with paradoxical anal sphincter contraction; type II, inadequate generation of
propulsive force and paradoxical contraction or inadequate relaxation of the
anal sphincters; and type III, generation of appropriate intrarectal pressure
with insufficient anal sphincter relaxation (Figure 3.5). Although each type of
dyssynergia has a different underlying mechanism, the outcomes are the same:
an inability to evacuate stool [3, 4]. Figure 3.6 illustrates the recto-anal

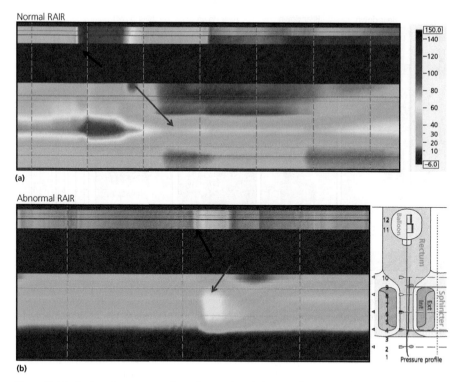

Figure 3.6 Isobaric color contour plots of normal and abnormal recto-anal inhibitory reflexes (RAIRs). (a) As the intrarectal pressure increases (black arrow), the internal anal sphincter reflexively relaxes (red arrow). This is a normal response. (b) As the intrarectal pressure increases (black arrow), there is no relaxation of the internal anal sphincter (red arrow). This is an inappropriate response.

inhibitory reflex. Ballon distension of the rectum stimulates reflex inhibition of the internal anal sphincter. The reflexive inhibition is impaired in Hirschsprung's disease.

Motility testing

Historically, physicians have used barium transit, nuclear scintigraphy, hydrogen breath testing, radio-opaque marker studies, and manometry to evaluate GI motility. Manometric testing with water-perfused assemblies has now been replaced by high-resolution solid-state manometric catheter recording. The advantages of this new technology include greater temporal and spatial fidelity, sophisticated automated data analysis, portability, and color contour topographic depictions of pressure data that make data interpretation easier. In addition, a wireless motility capsule, SmartPill (Given Imaging Ltd., Yokneam, Israel), has been developed that allows evaluation of gastric, small intestinal, colonic, and whole gut transit times. This capsule contains an array of sensors

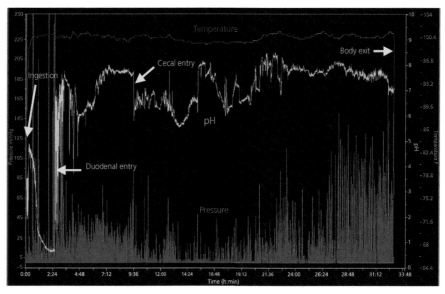

Figure 3.7 Wireless motility capsule tracing depicting simultaneous recordings of intraluminal temperature, pH, and pressure. (a) Gastric transit time: This is measured from the time the capsule is ingested until the time it enters the duodenum. This is best evaluated via the pH tracings (green lines). Entry into the duodenum is characterized by a large increase in pH, indicating a shift from the acidic milieu of the stomach to the alkalinized small intestine. (b) Small intestinal transit time: This is measured from the time the capsule enters the duodenum to the time it enters the cecum. This occurs when there is a decrease of at least 1 pH unit lasting more than 10 min and occurring greater than 30 min after entry of the capsule into the small intestine. The decrease in pH is believed secondary to acidic fermentation of digestive matter by colonic flora. This is best assessed by the pH tracings (green lines). (c) Colon transit time: This is measured from the time the capsule enters the cecum to the time it exits the body. The exit time can be determined using the blue lines. The temperature will remain stable throughout the study until the capsule is expelled from the body which will be characterized by a precipitous decrease in temperature correlating to the temperature of the water in the toilet basin. (d) Whole gut transit time: This is calculated from the time of ingestion until the capsule is passed as represented by the rapid decrease in temperature which correlates to passage of the capsule.

that simultaneously measure intraluminal pH, pressure, and temperature, allowing radiation-free regional transit time assessment (Figure 3.7). Comparative studies have demonstrated a reasonable correlation between data obtained with this device and data from conventional motility tests, including gastric and small bowel scintigraphy, and colonic radio-opaque markers. The wireless capsule appears most useful in the diagnosis of disorders causing global GI dysmotility, including scleroderma and amyloidosis, and for assessment of regional transit in patients with delayed gastric emptying and slow-transit constipation. The utility of pressure data collected throughout the GI tract with this technology has yet to be established [5].

Multiple choice questions

1 The abnormality that best describes the pathogenesis of diabetic gastroparesis is:
   A Enteric neuropathy associated with increased transient lower esophageal sphincter relaxation
   B Visceral myopathy affecting intestinal transit
   C Hypoglycemia-associated delayed gastric emptying
   D Central nervous system defect resulting in increased satiety
   E Autonomic neuropathy-associated impairment of gastric emptying

2 You are consulted to see a 58-year-old male with abdominal pain and distension. His symptoms began abrupted 4 days ago following an uneventful hip replacement. He has not moved his bowels or passed flatus since the surgery. On exam, he appears mildly uncomfortable and is afebrile with a pulse of 88. His abdomen is markedly distended and tympanitic with mild diffuse tenderness to palpation. A KUB demonstrates a diffusely and markedly distended colon filled with air with a cecal diameter of 12 cm. A gastrograffin enema documents patency of the rectum and sigmoid with colonic dilation. Appropriate therapy at this point would include which of the following pharmacologic agents:
   A 5HT3 antagonist
   B 5HT4 antagonist
   C Acetylcholinesterase inhibitor
   D Acetylcholine receptor antagonist
   E Opioid agonist

3 Hirschsprung's disease is caused by which of the following?
   A Impaired segmental transit of stool through the colon
   B Deficiency of excitatory neuronal innervation of the rectum
   C Deficiency of inhibitory neuronal innervation of the distal colon and rectum
   D Impaired relaxation of the external anal sphincter
   E Impaired contractions due to colonic dilation

4 Which statement is true?
   A The majority of the parasympathetic fibers innervating the GI tract originate in the spinal cord.
   B Parasympathetic innervations of the GI tract is indirect via the Enteric Nervous System
   C Sympathetic innervations generally stimulates motor and secretory activities in the GI tract
   D Parasympathetic innervations generally inhibits motor and secretory activities in the GI tract

5 A 56 year old male had a vagotomy for peptic ulcer disease twenty years ago. A nuclear medicine emptying study would most likely show?
   A Delayed solid and liquid emptying from the stomach.
   B Delayed liquid but normal solid emptying from the stomach.
   C Delayed solid and accelerated liquid emptying from the stomach.
   D Delayed liquid but accelerated solid emptying from the stomach.
   E Accelerated liquid and solid emptying

6 Which of the following is not a factor responsible for anal continence?
   A Tonic contractions of the puborectalis muscle
   B The external anal sphincter
   C The internal anal sphincter
   D Pudendal nerve innervation of the external anal sphincter
   E Sympathetic and parasympathetic stimulation of the internal anal sphincter

7 Local peristaltic reflexes in the GI tract are contained within the ENS and are characterized by?
   A Acetylcholine and Substance P exciting motor neurons above a food bolus
   B Nitric oxide and VIP exciting motor neurons above a food bolus
   C Acetylcholine and Substance P exciting motor neurons below a food bolus
   D Nitric oxide and VIP inhibiting motor neurons above a food bolus

8 Concerning the Migratory Motor Complex which statement is true?
  A Phase 2 propels gastric residue into the duodenum
  B Is stimulated immediately after eating
  C During phase 3 bacteria and residual food move from the small bowel into the colon
  D During phase 3 the pylorus pressure is elevated to inhibit gastric emptying.
  E Is inhibited by the hormone Motilin
9 (Pick the wrong answer) In the esophagus
  A Each swallow is normally followed by both segmental and peristaltic contractions
  B Both gut smooth muscle and striated muscle are stimulated by acetylcholine
  C Local stimulus can trigger a myogenic secondary peristaltic wave
  D Esophageal contractions can push swallowed material through the LES without the assistance of gravity
  E Esophageal spasms can cause chest pains that are very difficult to distinguish from those or coronary artery disease
10 Concerning Gastric Motility – all are true *except*:
  A The fundus is characterized by receptive relaxation which is mediated by NO and VIP.
  B Liquids empty faster than solids
  C Has a gastric basal electrical rate (BER) is 12 cycles/minute
  D When the pacemaker potentials (slow waves) are linked to action potentials of a great enough threshold muscle contractions occur
  E The pacemaker electrical activity of the stomach is generated by the Interstital cells of Cajal

References

1 Goyal, R.K. and Hirano, I. (1996) Mechanisms of disease: the enteric nervous system, *The New England Journal of Medicine*, **334**, 1106–1115.
2 Goyal and Shaker GI Motility Online. www.nature.com/gimo/index.html (accessed September 22, 2013).
3 Barucha, A.E. (2006) Pelvic floor: anatomy and function. *Neurogastroenterology and Motility*, **18**, 507–519.
4 Rao, S.S.C. (2007) Constipation: evaluation and treatment of colonic and anorectal motility disorders. *Gastrointestinal Endoscopy Clinics of North America*, **36**, 687–711.
5 Tran, K., Brun, R. and Kuo, B. (2012) Evaluation of regional and whole gut motility using the wireless motility capsule: relevance in clinical practice. *Therapeutic Advances in Gastroenterology*, **5** (4), 249–260.

Answers

1 E
2 C
3 C
4 B
5 C
6 E
7 A
8 C
9 A
10 C

CHAPTER 4

Gastrointestinal immunology and ecology

Shehzad Z. Sheikh[1] & Scott E. Plevy[2]

[1] Division of Gastroenterology and Hepatology, University of North Carolina School of Medicine, Chapel Hill, NC, USA
[2] Departments of Medicine, Microbiology and Immunology, University of North Carolina School of Medicine, Chapel Hill, NC, USA

Introduction

The primary function of the immune system is to protect the individual from pathogens. Physical and chemical barriers limit the ability of harmful molecules to interact with the immune system outside the GI tract. The GI mucosal immune system is unique in that it is constantly in contact with the external environment. All ingested substances contain foreign antigens capable of eliciting an immune response, and, therefore, GI immune cells must be able to distinguish between potentially harmful and harmless antigens to avoid a constant state of gut inflammation. The general strategy of the mucosal immune system to accomplish this goal is suppression or downregulation of immune responses. This strategy is facilitated or characterized by several unique features of mucosal immunity: secretory IgA production, suppression of IgG and IgM responses, chronic controlled (physiologic) inflammation, and oral tolerance.

Failure of this tightly regulated system may lead to chronic uncontrolled mucosal inflammation as exemplified by the IBD. A working hypothesis of IBD pathogenesis is that there is an inappropriate inflammatory immune response to enteric microbes that normally coexist in a mutually beneficial relationship with their human hosts.

The anatomy of the mucosal immune system

All mucosal surfaces and their associated lymphoid tissue are part of a common immune system. Each mucosal surface is formed by a layer of epithelium overlying a lamina propria containing loosely organized lymphoid tissue that, in the GI tract, is referred to as the gut-associated lymphoid tissue (GALT) [1]. The length and enormous surface area of the GI tract make it the largest lymphoid organ of the body, containing greater than 10^{12} lymphocytes and more antibody

Gastrointestinal Anatomy and Physiology: The Essentials, First Edition. Edited by John F. Reinus and Douglas Simon.
© 2014 John Wiley & Sons, Ltd. Published 2014 by John Wiley & Sons, Ltd.
www.wiley.com/go/reinus/gastro/anatomy

than is found at any other site [1]. The GI epithelium is a single layer of columnar cells covered by an extracellular glycocalyx composed of complex glycoproteins and mucins. This glycocalyx coat is an important physical barrier to potential pathogens; microbial organisms become trapped within it and are passed in stool. The epithelium itself is a second level of physical protection: epithelial cell membranes prevent most bacteria and viruses from reaching underlying lymphoid tissue [2]. Tight junctions joining adjacent cells are a third level of physical protection. These tight junctions maintain the integrity of the epithelial barrier and exclude macromolecules and pathogens [2]. Inflammation may compromise the integrity of tight junctions, resulting in a "leaky" epithelium that allows luminal contents to reach the lamina propria [3]. Indeed, several IBD susceptibility genes may affect intestinal epithelial permeability [4].

Sites of mucosal immune–microbial interactions

Interactions between commensal bacteria, antigens, and immune cells occur at distinct sites in the GI tract, such as PPs [5]. PPs are organized GI tract structures analogous to lymph nodes in which naïve T and B cells first encounter antigens from the intestinal lumen [5]. PPs are covered by M cells, specialized intestinal epithelial cells (IECs) that lack surface microvilli or glycocalyxes [6]. These cells facilitate passage of antigens, especially large particulate antigens, bacteria, and viruses, from the gut lumen to T cells in PPs and mesenteric lymph nodes. Antigens pass through M cells intact and subsequently are taken up by dedicated antigen-presenting cells (APCs) (dendritic cells (DCs) and macrophages) in the M-cell pocket. The APCs carry them to T-cell zones in PPs or mesenteric lymph nodes where they generate an immune response [5, 6]. Activated T cells in the GALT then circulate back to the lamina propria via the efferent lymph and the blood stream (Figure 4.1).

Luminal antigens also interact with the mucosal space through M-cell-independent pathways mediated by DCs from the lamina propria [7]. These specialized DCs extend dendrites into the lumen and sample its content, much in the same manner as M cells do [8]. Gut columnar epithelial cells also can process antigens, albeit far less efficiently than do dedicated APCs (Figure 4.1) [6].

Secretory IgA

Secretory IgA, a unique form of antibody found in mucosal secretions, is an important effector of mucosal immunity. While IgG is the most abundant immunoglobulin in serum, IgA is the most abundant in secretions. IgA is secreted by terminally differentiated B cells (plasma cells) in the lamina propria that recognize antigens from the intestinal lumen [9]. Secretory IgA differs from IgA in serum. In serum,

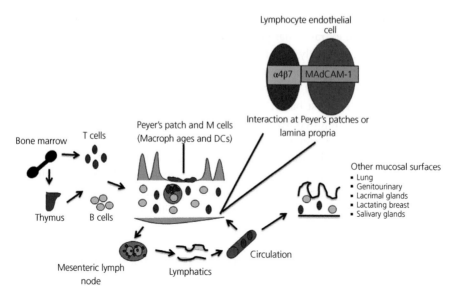

Figure 4.1 The gut immune system. Interactions between commensal bacteria, antigens, and immune cells occur at PPs and isolated follicles, where M cells in the follicle-associated epithelium translocate bacterial antigens from the lumen to the dome region beneath the follicle-associated epithelium. Immature myeloid DCs and macrophages encounter and process antigen, differentiate into mature DCs, and migrate to T-cell zones in PP or to mesenteric lymph nodes to activate T cells. The organized GALT serves as the source of the activated effector cells, which populate the intervening mucosa; cells leave via efferent lymph, enter the blood stream, and migrate back to the lamina propria. Lymphocyte trafficking to the intestine is directed by adhesion receptors.

IgA exists as a monomer and is not a particularly useful antibody, whereas in secretions, it exists as a dimer and is coated with a highly specialized 55-kD glycoprotein called secretory component that is derived from cleavage of the polymeric Ig receptor [9].

The polymeric Ig receptor and secretory component serve two purposes. First, they transport IgA from the lamina propria to the gut lumen. The polymeric Ig receptor is expressed on the basolateral aspect of the IEC and binds only to dimeric IgA or multimeric IgM. IgA complexed with the receptor is actively transported within vesicles to the apical epithelial cell membrane. The Ig receptor is partially cleaved within the vesicle, leaving a portion remaining in association with IgA as the secretory component. The vesicle then fuses with the apical epithelial cell membrane and the secretory component–IgA complex is released into the lumen. Within the lumen, secretory component serves a second function: it shields the secretory IgA molecule from degradation by intraluminal proteases and gastric acid. Secretory IgA and IgM are the only antibodies that can bind secretory component and thereby withstand the harsh environment of the GI tract [9].

In the lamina propria and gut lumen, secretory IgA has a passive function. As IgA does not activate complement or bind Fc receptors, it does not mediate inflammatory responses. Rather, secretory IgA directed against microbial antigens blocks their binding to the epithelium, thereby preventing infection [9]. Secretory IgA also can agglutinate bacteria and viruses into large complexes that are trapped in the mucus barrier and passed in stool, sputum, and vaginal secretions.

Secretory IgA is reabsorbed in the distal small intestine and reused. IgA complexed with antigen is taken up in the distal ileum, enters the portal circulation, and travels to the liver where sinusoidal Kupffer cells remove and destroy the antigen, releasing free secretory IgA. Bile duct epithelial cells also express the polymeric Ig receptor on their basolateral surfaces and actively transport secretory IgA into bile. Because bile flows into the intestine, this IgA ultimately can be reused against pathogens in the GI tract [9].

B cells in PPs become committed to produce IgA: under the influence of transforming growth factor beta (TGFβ), an IgA switch factor, PP B cells that make and express surface IgM switch their genetic program to transcribe and produce IgA [5]. These cells then migrate to mesenteric lymph nodes, enter the thoracic duct, and ultimately reach the systemic circulation. IgA B cells enter the LP from the circulation at various mucosal sites where they differentiate into plasma cells that produce IgA. One key site is the mammary gland, where secretory IgA plasma cells secrete IgA into breast milk. In countries where intestinal parasites and bacterial diarrheal illnesses are endemic, this is the major means of passively immunizing the infant: as IgA survives in the gut, it binds parasites and bacteria in the lumen and prevents disease [9].

Cells of the mucosal immune system

The unique nature of MALT is further exemplified by the distinct phenotypic and functional characteristics of its constituent immune cells. Several important cell types are found in PPs, such as IgA-secreting B cells, which already have been discussed. Here, we discuss the unique features of T cells in the epithelial space and LP, as well as DCs and macrophages, the professional APCs of the MALT.

Intraepithelial lymphocytes (IELs)
IELs are small cells located within the epithelium of mucosal surfaces. More than 98% express cluster of differentiation antigen 8 (CD8), a coreceptor for MHC class I molecules. When isolated, they resist activation through the T-cell receptor and barely proliferate, even in response to potent stimuli. IELs do not appear to travel in and out of the epithelium; rather epithelial cells grow over them as they

move from the crypt to the surface. The majority of studies suggest that IELs are *not* involved in immune responses against luminal pathogens. Instead, they appear to be engaged in cytotoxicity, including alloreactive virus-specific and spontaneous cytotoxicity, activities consistent with an immune surveillance or first-line-of-defense role. Subsets of IELs provide B-cell help, play a role in the maintenance of oral tolerance, and regulate epithelial cell function [10].

Virtually, all IELs express the selective integrin αEβ7. Its ligand on the IEC is E-cadherin, which is involved in cell signaling and cytoskeletal rearrangement. Unlike related integrins, it does not appear that αEβ7 is a homing molecule [10].

Lamina propria lymphocytes (LPL)

Several types of immune cells are found in the lamina propria. IgA-producing plasma cells predominate, but over half of this population is comprised of T cells, B cells, macrophages, and DCs. *Controlled* inflammation is an important characteristic of the LP [2]. The abundance of activated lymphocytes and APCs in the GALT would signify chronic inflammatory disease if present in other organs [1]. Control of inflammation in the gut is the result of regulatory mechanisms that prevent deleterious inflammatory responses to normal luminal contents, such as dietary constituents and resident nonpathogenic microbes. For example, like IELs, lamina propria T cells express an activated–memory phenotype and do not proliferate in response to T-cell receptor ligands. In contrast, they express the mucosal addressin, α4β7. This addressin recognizes a gut-specific adhesion molecule, MadCAM-1, expressed solely by GI vascular endothelium [11, 12]. Hence, this interaction mediates specific homing of leukocytes to the intestine (Figure 4.2). Lamina propria T cells undergo spontaneous apoptosis at higher rates *in vitro* and *in vivo* than do peripheral blood lymphocytes [13]. Patients with IBD have defects in the mechanisms that regulate T-cell apoptosis [14].

Mucosal T cells: Inflammatory and regulatory subsets

Cytokines elaborated by CD4-positive helper T cells in the lamina propria play a key role in the regulation of intestinal immune responses. T-helper-1 (Th1) cells produce the inflammatory cytokines interferon-γ (Ifn-γ) and interleukin-2 (IL-2), which are necessary for eradication of intracellular pathogens and the development of long-term immunity against these infectious agents [15]. Chronic intestinal inflammation results from persistence of unchecked mucosal Th1 cell responses. Crohn's disease is a typical human Th1-mediated chronic inflammatory disorder, characterized by mucosal granuloma formation (the histological hallmark of a Th1 immune response), increased expression of Ifn-γ, and increased expression of IL-12 and IL-18, two cytokines necessary to development of a Th1 immune response [15]. Th2 cells develop primarily in response to helminth and allergen exposure; IL-4, IL-5, and IL-13 are hallmark

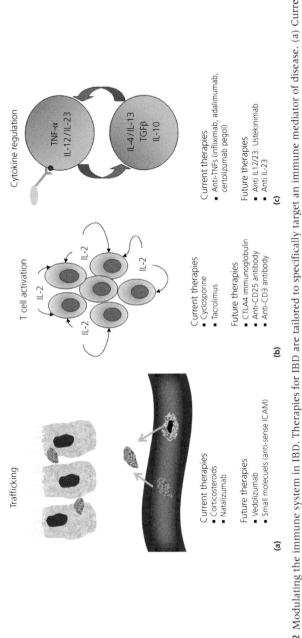

Figure 4.2 Modulating the immune system in IBD. Therapies for IBD are tailored to specifically target an immune mediator of disease. (a) Current therapies that target immune cell trafficking to inflamed intestinal mucosa include corticosteroids and natalizumab (antibody that blocks interaction between integrin α4 on the leukocyte and MAdCAM1 on the endothelial cell). Emerging therapies include inhibition of integrin α4β7 and MAdCAM1 that occurs specifically in the vascular endothelium of the intestines and other small molecules, for example, silencing RNAs targeting adhesions molecules in the vascular endothelium(b) T-cell activation is the target of widely used immunomodulator therapy in IBD that includes azathioprine, 6-mercaptopurine, methotrexate, cyclosporine, and tacrolimus. Clinical trials for antibodies directed toward T cells (CD3) and subset populations (CD23, Tregs) are being conducted; (c) the monoclonal antibodies to tumor necrosis factor (TNF) (infliximab, a mouse–human chimeric antibody; adalimumab, a humanized recombinant antibody to TNF; and certolizumab pegol, a Fab fragment of a humanized anti-TNF alpha monoclonal antibody that is attached to polyethylene glycol to increase its half-life in circulation) are FDA-approved biological therapies for IBD. Future therapies target the IL-12 and IL-23 axis.

cytokines produced by Th2 cells. These cytokines aid B-cell antibody production and, in the mucosal immune system, also are involved in host defense against extracellular helminthic parasites [15]. Th17 cells are specific effectors that play a role in host defense against extracellular bacteria and fungi [16]. In contrast to Crohn's disease, early descriptive studies of human ulcerative colitis patients demonstrated colonic Th2 cytokines [17]. Human T-cell biology is complex, however, and when characterizing intestinal T-cell responses in heterogeneous disease populations, the Th1–Th2 classification that may be relevant in mice is overly simplistic.

Several important regulatory T (Treg)-cell populations restrain inflammatory mucosal Th1 immune responses in normally controlled inflammation. For example, Treg cells downregulate inflammatory responses [18]. Treg cells make the anti-inflammatory cytokines IL-10 and TGFβ, which are important mediators of mucosal homeostasis [18]. TGFβ also mediates mucosal healing and fibrogenesis and is necessary to IgA production. Treg cells mediate the phenomenon of oral tolerance, which is a state of immune unresponsiveness to intestinal luminal antigens [18]. IBD patients lose tolerance to their own enteric bacteria, demonstrating the importance of these Treg-cell subsets in maintaining controlled inflammation.

Mucosal macrophages and dendritic cells

Macrophages and DCs are essential to innate immunity against enteric microbes. Intestinal macrophages represent the largest pool of tissue monocytes in the human body and are critical to immune interactions with the enteric microbiota. In comparison to other macrophages, intestinal macrophages express different phenotypic markers and efficiently eradicate intracellular bacteria, but do not mount potent inflammatory responses [19].

Both macrophages and DCs play a crucial role in shaping the T-cell immune response through cognate interactions with T cells and by producing cytokines, some induced by bacteria. They can induce an inflammatory Th1 or Th17 immune response through production of IL-12 and IL-23, respectively, or divert the immune response toward a regulatory pathway through production of IL-10 and TGFβ [20]. DCs are the most potent APCs for induction of primary T-cell responses. DCs that induce Treg-cell populations predominate in PPs [20]. A distinct population of DCs that transports fragments of apoptotic IECs to the T-cell regions of mesenteric lymph nodes has recently been described and may serve the primary function of inducing naive T-cell tolerance to self-IEC antigens [7, 21]. The importance of functional adaptations of macrophages and DCs in this unique environment is best illustrated by failure of these homeostatic mechanisms in the development of IBD [22, 19] (Figure 4.2).

Intestinal epithelial cells

The intestinal epithelium plays a critical role in mucosal immune homeostasis. IECs line the mucosal surface, acting as a physical barrier to invasion by pathogens, including organisms that initiate specific and nonspecific host immune responses. IECs also play an active role in initiating immune responses by elaborating cytokines, chemokines, and other inflammatory mediators, some of which promote migration of T cells to the GI tract [3]. They are one component of a complex signaling system characterized as a "trialogue" among the intestinal microbiota, the intestinal epithelium, and the GALT [23].

Infection of human IECs by enteroinvasive bacteria increases expression and secretion of a number of proinflammatory cytokines, including chemokines that are potent chemoattractants for acute inflammatory cells [24]. In response to pathogens, IECs also express inflammatory cytokines that recruit and activate leukocytes and macrophages, whereas they produce activated TGFβ in healthy individuals [24]. Thus, inflammatory gene expression by IECs is an important component of the innate immune response against enteric pathogens [25].

Interactions between noninvasive bacteria and IECs are also important, profoundly affecting IEC gene expression, differentiation, growth, and initiation of immune responses [3]. Resident bacteria induce IEC gene expression required for normal intestinal development and function [24]. Deviations from this normal program as a result of transient bacterial colonization, altered host genetics, or both may initiate inflammatory gene expression and chronic intestinal inflammation [25].

As mentioned previously, M cells sample particulate antigens and intact microorganisms in PPs [5]. They are, however, inefficient at taking up soluble proteins [6]. IECs may play a role in sampling luminal antigen by expression of MHC class II molecules that take up soluble proteins at the apical cell membrane and transport them to the basolateral cell membrane. Despite expression of MHC class II antigens, normal IECs appear to selectively activate CD8+ suppressor T cells, and, therefore, antigen presentation by IECs may downregulate inflammatory T cells or may generate regulatory, suppressor, or anti-inflammatory T-cell subsets [7, 23, 26]. This may help to explain the inhibitory phenomena of controlled inflammation and oral tolerance [27].

Immunosuppression in the GI tract: Oral tolerance

Oral tolerance, which can be viewed as the opposite of immunization, is a hallmark of the gut's controlled immune response. Soluble antigens administered orally, instead of subcutaneously or intramuscularly, induce antigen-specific unresponsiveness [28]. Oral tolerance is likely important in preventing immune responses to dietary antigens and enteric flora [29]. As oral tolerance is a potent physiologic mechanism for suppression of immune responses, induction of oral tolerance may be of therapeutic benefit in autoimmune diseases. In theory, an autoantigen can be used to induce Treg cells that attenuate local inflammation because although induction of oral tolerance is antigen specific, the mechanism of tolerance (generation of TGFβ) is not. Therefore, it may be possible to use an antigen located in proximity to an autoantigen to trigger TGFβ secretion that inhibits the autoantigen response. This phenomenon has been termed bystander suppression [30].

The enteric ecosystem

The GI tract is home to a dense, diverse, and dynamic bacterial ecosystem that is critical to mucosal immune homeostasis. The commensal flora of the gut is estimated to be comprised of 500–1000 distinct bacterial species, with the total number of bacteria approaching 10^{14} cells and containing 100 times as many genes as the human genome [31].

This enteric microbiota is important to human health. Commensal bacteria are essential to the preservation of the integrity of the mucosal barrier, and interruption of this barrier has been implicated in the pathophysiology of IBD [25]. The enteric microbiota also modulates the intestinal immune system and is essential to the maturation of the GALT, secretion of IgA, and production of antimicrobial peptides [32]. Additionally, gut floras have metabolic capabilities lacking in the host, such as fermentation of indigestible fiber, and can help the host by degrading otherwise indigestible dairy products. Importantly, the microbiota can modulate host gene expression, and conversely, host metabolism influences the microbial environment.

Conclusion

The intestinal epithelial barrier and specialized immune cell populations of the gut differentiate pathogenic from beneficial commensal bacteria and, therefore, are essential to maintaining immune homeostasis. Given its potentially hostile environment, an overall tone of suppression is a necessary adaptation of the GI immune system. Defects in intestinal permeability and regulatory immune cell populations and alterations in the microbial ecosystem may lead to inappropriate immune responses in an otherwise immune-tolerant environment. A vicious cycle can ensue in which increased intestinal permeability allows translocation of large amounts of luminal antigen that amplifies ongoing mucosal inflammation and causes IBD. Thus, IBD results from an inappropriately directed inflammatory response to the enteric microbiota in a genetically susceptible host [31] (Figure 4.2).

Multiple choice questions

1 Based on the functional characteristics of the mucosal immune system, which of these new therapies for inflammatory bowel disease does not make theoretic sense?
   A Antibodies that block interleukin-23
   B Altering the intestinal bacterial flora with probiotic bacteria
   C Antibodies that block the alpha4beta7–MadCAM-1 interaction
   D Antibodies that block TGFbeta
   E Antibodies that prevent T-cell activation

2 Sensing of microbes and microbial antigens at the mucosal surface occurs through a series of "mucosal monitors" which include all of the following except:
   A Mesenteric lymph nodes
   B Spleen
   C Peyer's patches
   D Lamina propria antigen-presenting cells
   E Intestinal epithelial cells

3 All the following statements concerning the GI immunology and disease are correct *except*:
   A M cells in the lumen sample antigen and pass the antigen to the Peyer's patches below.
   B Peyer's patches are the only organized immune cells in the GI tract.
   C Inflammatory bowel disease is considered a disease failure of the GI tract immune system to downregulate.
   D Antigens are taken up by M cells, and the M cell presents those antigens to lymphocytes in Peyer's patches.
   E Secretory component facilitates transport of IgA from the lamina propria to the lumen and facilitates the enterohepatic circulation of IgA.

4 Which statement is false:
   A In the serum, IgA exists as a dimer and in the gut, it is a monomer.
   B Secretory component binds to IgA and facilitates its movement into the lumen of the GI tract.
   C Secretory component protects IgA from degradation by luminal enzymes.
   D The secretory IgA (sIgA) binds to bacteria and viruses in the GI tract.
   E After sIgA binds to its antigen, the complex is taken up in the terminal ileum, travels to the liver, and is taken up by Kupffer cells.

5 The ability to generate oral tolerance to a specific antigen depends upon:
   A The age of the host
   B The genetic background
   C The solubility of the antigen
   D The dose of the antigen
   E The chemical composition of the host (protein vs. carbohydrate vs. lipid)
   F All of the above

References

1 Macdonald, T.T. and Monteleone, G. (2005) Immunity, inflammation, and allergy in the gut. *Science*, **307**, 1920–1925.
2 Pearson, C., Uhlig, H.H. and Powrie, F. (2012) Lymphoid microenvironments and innate lymphoid cells in the gut. *Trends in Immunology*, **33**, 289–296.
3 Schulzke, J.D., Ploeger, S., Amasheh, M. *et al.* (2009) Epithelial tight junctions in intestinal inflammation. *Annals of the New York Academy of Sciences*, **1165**, 294–300.

4 Franke, A., McGovern, D.P., Barrett, J.C. *et al.* (2010) Genome-wide meta-analysis increases to 71 the number of confirmed Crohn's disease susceptibility loci. *Nature Genetics*, **42**, 1118–1125.

5 Craig, S.W. and Cebra, J.J. (1971) Peyer's patches: an enriched source of precursors for IgA-producing immunocytes in the rabbit. *The Journal of Experimental Medicine*, **134**, 188–200.

6 Kyd, J.M. and Cripps, A.W. (2008) Functional differences between M cells and enterocytes in sampling luminal antigens. *Vaccine*, **26**, 6221–6224.

7 Rescigno, M., Urbano, M., Valzasina, B. *et al.* (2001) Dendritic cells express tight junction proteins and penetrate gut epithelial monolayers to sample bacteria. *Nature Immunology*, **2**, 361–367.

8 Chieppa, M., Rescigno, M., Huang, A.Y. and Germain R.N. (2006) Dynamic imaging of dendritic cell extension into the small bowel lumen in response to epithelial cell TLR engagement. *The Journal of Experimental Medicine*, **203**, 2841–2852.

9 Macpherson, A.J., Geuking, M.B. and McCoy, K.D. (2012) Homeland security: IgA immunity at the frontiers of the body. *Trends in Immunology*, **33**, 160–167.

10 Cheroutre, H., Lambolez, F. and Mucida, D. (2011) The light and dark sides of intestinal intraepithelial lymphocytes. *Nature Reviews Immunology*, **11**, 445–456.

11 Hart, A.L., Ng, S.C., Mann, E. *et al.* (1969) Homing of immune cells: role in homeostasis and intestinal inflammation. *Inflammatory Bowel Disease*, **16**, 1969–1977.

12 Gorfu, G., Rivera-Nieves, J. and Ley, K. (2009) Role of beta7 integrins in intestinal lymphocyte homing and retention. *Current Molecular Medicine*, **9**, 836–850.

13 Neurath, M.F., Finotto, S., Fuss, I. *et al.* (2001) Regulation of T-cell apoptosis in inflammatory bowel disease: to die or not to die, that is the mucosal question. *Trends in Immunology*, **22**, 21–26.

14 Lugering, A., Lebiedz, P., Koch, S. and Kucharzik, T. (2006) Apoptosis as a therapeutic tool in IBD? *Annals of the New York Academy of Sciences*, **1072**, 62–77.

15 O'Garra, A., McEvoy, L.M. and Zlotnik, A. (1998) T-cell subsets: chemokine receptors guide the way. *Current Biology*, **8**, R646–R649.

16 Harrington, L.E., Mangan, P.R. and Weaver, C.T. (2006) Expanding the effector CD4 T-cell repertoire: the Th17 lineage. *Current Opinion in Immunology*, **18**, 349–356.

17 Niessner, M. and Volk, B.A. (1995) Altered Th1/Th2 cytokine profiles in the intestinal mucosa of patients with inflammatory bowel disease as assessed by quantitative reversed transcribed polymerase chain reaction (RT-PCR). *Clinical and Experimental Immunology*, **101**, 428–435.

18 Izcue, A., Coombes, J.L. and Powrie, F. (2006) Regulatory T cells suppress systemic and mucosal immune activation to control intestinal inflammation. *Immunological Reviews*, **212**, 256–271.

19 Kamada, N., Hisamatsu, T., Okamoto, S. *et al.* (2008) Unique CD14 intestinal macrophages contribute to the pathogenesis of Crohn disease via IL-23/IFN-gamma axis. *The Journal of Clinical Investigation*, **118**, 2269–2280.

20 Coombes JL, Powrie F. Dendritic cells in intestinal immune regulation. *Nat Rev Immunol* 2008;8:435–46.

21 Coombes, J.L., Siddiqui, K.R., Arancibia-Carcamo, C.V. *et al.* (2007) A functionally specialized population of mucosal CD103+ DCs induces Foxp3+ regulatory T cells via a TGF-beta and retinoic acid-dependent mechanism. *Journal of Experimental Medicine*, **204**, 1757–1764.

22 Glocker, E.O., Kotlarz, D. and Boztug, K. *et al.* (2009) Inflammatory bowel disease and mutations affecting the interleukin-10 receptor. *The New England Journal of Medicine*, **361**, 2033–2045.

23 Rimoldi, M., Chieppa, M., Salucci, V. *et al.* (2005) Intestinal immune homeostasis is regulated by the crosstalk between epithelial cells and dendritic cells. *Nature Immunology*, **6**, 507–514.

24 Rakoff-Nahoum, S. and Medzhitov, R. (2008) Innate immune recognition of the indigenous microbial flora. *Mucosal Immunology*, **1**(Suppl 1), S10–S14.

25 McGuckin, M.A., Eri, R., Simms, LA. *et al.* (2009). Intestinal barrier dysfunction in inflammatory bowel diseases. *Inflammatory Bowel Diseases*, **15**, 100–113.

26 Guy-Grand, D., Cerf-Bensussan, N., Malissen, B. *et al.* (1991) Two gut intraepithelial CD8+ lymphocyte populations with different T cell receptors: a role for the gut epithelium in T cell differentiation. *Journal of Experimental Medicine*, **173**, 471–481.

27 Xavier, R.J. and Podolsky, D.K. (2007) Unravelling the pathogenesis of inflammatory bowel disease. *Nature*, **448**, 427–434.

28 Pabst, O. and Mowat, A.M. (2012) Oral tolerance to food protein. *Mucosal Immunology*, **5**, 232–239.

29 Miron, N. and Cristea, V. (2012) Enterocytes: active cells in tolerance to food and microbial antigens in the gut. *Clinical & Experimental Immunology*, **167**, 405–412.

30 Molloy, M.J., Bouladoux, N. and Belkaid, Y. (2012) Intestinal microbiota: shaping local and systemic immune responses. *Seminars in Immunology*, **24**, 58–66.

31 Sartor, R.B. (2006) Mechanisms of disease: pathogenesis of Crohn's disease and ulcerative colitis. *Nature Clinical Practice Gastroenterology & Hepatology*, **3**, 390–407.

32 Mantis, N.J., Rol, N. and Corthesy, B. (2011) Secretory IgA's complex roles in immunity and mucosal homeostasis in the gut. *Mucosal Immunology*, **4**, 603–611.

Answers

1 D
2 B
3 D
4 A
5 F

CHAPTER 5

Gastric physiology

Mitchell L. Schubert

Virginia Commonwealth University's Medical College of Virginia, Richmond, VA, USA
Division of Gastroenterology, McGuire Veterans Affairs Medical Center, Richmond, VA, USA

Overview

The stomach is an active reservoir that stores, grinds, and slowly dispenses partially digested food into the intestine for further digestion and absorption. One of its main functions is the secretion of hydrochloric acid. Gastric acid facilitates the digestion of protein by converting pepsinogen to the active proteolytic enzyme, pepsin. Acid also facilitates the absorption of iron, calcium, vitamin B_{12}, and some medications (e.g., thyroxin and ketoconazole) and prevents bacterial overgrowth, enteric infection, and, possibly, community-acquired pneumonia, spontaneous bacterial peritonitis, and IgE-mediated food allergy [1–9]. Too much acid, however, may overwhelm mucosal defense mechanisms and cause ulceration of the esophagus, stomach, and duodenum, as well as malabsorption.

The gastric mucosa secretes pepsinogen, lipase, intrinsic factor, electrolytes, and mucins, in addition to a variety of neurocrine, paracrine, and hormonal agents. Neurocrine agents (e.g., acetylcholine (ACh), gastrin-releasing peptide (GRP), vasoactive intestinal peptide (VIP), pituitary adenylate cyclase-activating polypeptide (PACAP) and calcitonin-gene related peptide (CGRP)) are released from nerve terminals and reach their targets via synaptic diffusion. Paracrine agents (e.g., histamine and somatostatin (SST)) are released from neuroendocrine cells in proximity to their targets and reach them via diffusion. Hormones (e.g., gastrin) are released into the circulation and reach their targets via the bloodstream.

Functional anatomy

The stomach consists of three anatomic (fundus, corpus or body, and antrum) and two functional (oxyntic- and pyloric-glandular mucosa) regions (Figure 5.1). There is debate as to whether the cardia, a transition zone of 0–9 mm between the squamous mucosa of the esophagus and the oxyntic mucosa of the fundus,

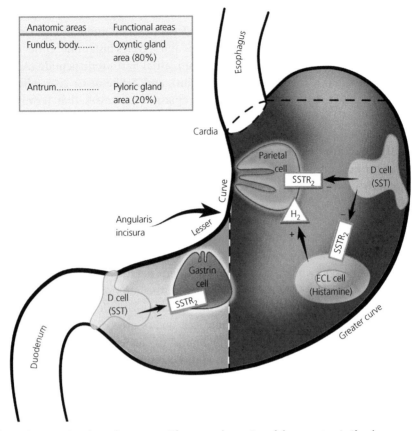

Figure 5.1 Functional gastric anatomy. The stomach consists of three anatomic (fundus, corpus or body, and antrum) and two functional (oxyntic and pyloric gland) areas. The hallmark of the oxyntic gland area is the parietal cell, whereas that of the pyloric gland area is the G or gastrin cell. SST-containing D cells are present in both functional areas. Their cytoplasmic processes terminate in the vicinity of acid-secreting parietal cells and histamine-secreting ECL cells in the oxyntic gland area (fundus and corpus) and gastrin-secreting G cells in the pyloric gland area (antrum). The functional correlate of this anatomic coupling is a tonic restraint exerted by SST on acid secretion that is exerted directly on the parietal cell as well as indirectly by inhibiting histamine and gastrin secretion. From Reference [10]. Reproduced with permission of Elsevier.

exists as a normal anatomic structure or develops as a result of gastroesophageal reflux. Autopsy and endoscopy studies suggest that the cardia is absent in over 50% of people [11].

Oxyntic mucosa, the hallmark of which is the oxyntic or parietal cell, lines 80% of the stomach (fundus and corpus). The gastric gland is divided into four regions: pit, isthmus, neck, and base. Stem and progenitor cells are located in the isthmus. Parietal cells reside in the middle regions but are able to migrate upwards and downwards. Parietal cells secrete hydrochloric acid and intrinsic factor. Chief cells reside in the base of the gland and secrete pepsinogen. Gastric glands contain a variety of neuroendocrine cell types, but the physiologic function of only some of their products has been discovered. The dominant endocrine cell is the enterochromaffin-like (ECL) cell that produces and secretes histamine. Other cells include enterochromaffin (EC) cells (serotonin, atrial natriuretic peptide (ANP), and adrenomedullin), D cells (SST and amylin), and A-like or Gr cells (ghrelin and obestatin) [12–16]. D cells possess cytoplasmic processes that terminate in the vicinity of parietal and ECL cells [14]. This anatomic feature allows tonic paracrine restraint of acid secretion by SST, that acts directly as well as indirectly through inhibition of histamine secretion [17] (Figure 5.1).

Pyloric mucosa, the hallmark of which is the gastrin or G cell, lines 20% of the stomach (antrum) (Figure 5.1). SST-containing D cells are also present in the pyloric mucosa where they exert a tonic paracrine restraint on gastrin secretion [18]. Pyloric glands contain chief cells (pepsinogen), EC cells (serotonin and ANP), A-like or Gr cells (ghrelin and obestatin), and endocrine cells containing orexin [19–21].

An extensive neural network, termed the enteric nervous system (ENS), innervates the stomach. The ENS, the third division of the autonomic nervous system (the other two being the sympathetic and parasympathetic), is composed of intrinsic neurons, that is, neurons whose cell bodies are contained within the gastric wall. Often referred to as the "little brain," the ENS contains as many neurons as the spinal cord and can function without central input [22]. It should be noted that the vagus nerve is mainly afferent and contains only 10–20% efferent fibers. The efferent fibers, which arise from the brain stem, are preganglionic and do not directly innervate gastric parietal or neuroendocrine cells; rather, they synapse with postganglionic intrinsic neurons of the ENS that contain a variety of transmitters, including ACh, GRP, VIP, and PACAP. The postganglionic neurons regulate secretion directly (e.g., ACh) and indirectly by modulating the secretion of gastrin from G cells (e.g., GRP), SST from D cells (e.g., ACh, GRP, VIP, and PACAP), and possibly histamine from ECL cells (e.g., PACAP) (Figure 5.2 and Figure 5.3).

Regulation of gastric acid secretion

The human stomach contains one billion parietal cells, each of which secretes hydrochloric acid at a concentration of approximately 160 mM or pH 0.8. In order to prevent acid from overwhelming mucosal defense mechanisms and causing tissue injury to the esophagus, stomach, and duodenum, acid secretion must be precisely regulated according to need. This is accomplished by a coordinated interaction among a variety of neural, hormonal, and paracrine pathways. These pathways can be activated by stimuli originating in the brain (cephalic phase) or reflexively by mechanical (e.g., distension) or chemical (e.g., amino acid, protein, and acid) stimuli originating in the stomach (gastric phase) after ingestion of a meal. The principal stimulants of acid secretion are (i) histamine,

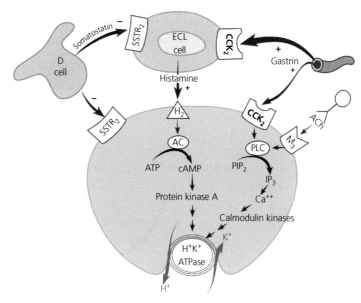

Figure 5.2 Model illustrating the receptors and transduction pathways regulating acid secretion by the parietal cell. The principal stimulants of acid secretion at the level of the parietal cell are histamine (paracrine), gastrin (hormonal), and ACh (neurocrine). Histamine, released from ECL cells, binds to H_2 receptors that activate AC and convert adenosine-5'-triphosphate (ATP) to adenosine 3',5'-cyclic monophosphate (cAMP). Increases in cAMP activate cAMP-dependent protein kinases (PKA) to phosphorylate intracellular proteins that ultimately elicit acid secretion. Gastrin, released from G cells, binds to CCK_2 receptors that activate phospholipase C (PLC) with conversion of phosphatidylinositol bisphosphate (PIP_2) to inositol trisphosphate (IP_3). IP_3, in turn, induces release of cytosolic calcium (Ca^{++}) with activation of calcium-dependent enzymes, such as calmodulin kinases, that ultimately elicit acid secretion. The acid stimulatory effects of gastrin, however, are currently thought to be mediated primarily by release of histamine from ECL cells (thick arrow). ACh, released from postganglionic intramural neurons, binds to M_3 receptors that are coupled to an increase in intracellular Ca^{++} via similar pathways described previously for gastrin. The intracellular cAMP- and calcium-dependent signaling systems activate downstream kinases that ultimately lead to fusion and activation of H^+K^+-ATPase, the proton pump. SST, released from oxyntic D cells, is the principal inhibitor of acid secretion. Acting via the $SSTR_2$ receptor, SST inhibits parietal cell secretion directly as well as indirectly by inhibiting histamine release from ECL cells. +, stimulatory; –, inhibitory. From Reference [10]. Reproduced with permission of Elsevier.

released from oxyntic ECL cells (paracrine); (ii) gastrin, released from antral G cells (hormonal); and (iii) ACh, released from postganglionic enteric neurons (neurocrine). These agents interact with specific receptors (H_2, cholecystokinin (CCK)$_2$, and M_3, respectively) on parietal cells that are coupled to two major signal transduction pathways: adenylate cyclase (AC) in the case of histamine and intracellular calcium in the case of gastrin and ACh. The main inhibitor of acid secretion is SST, released from oxyntic and pyloric D cells (paracrine).

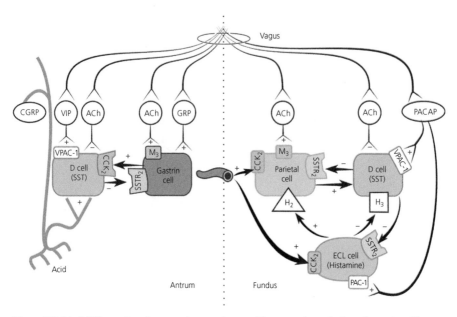

Figure 5.3 Model illustrating the neural, paracrine, and hormonal regulation of gastric acid secretion. Vagal efferent fibers synapse with intramural gastric cholinergic (ACh) and peptidergic (GRP, VIP, and PACAP) neurons. In the fundus and corpus (oxyntic mucosa), ACh neurons stimulate acid secretion directly (via M_3 receptors) as well as indirectly by inhibiting SST secretion (via M_2 and M_4 receptors), thus eliminating its restraint on parietal and histamine-containing ECL cells. In the antrum (pyloric mucosa), ACh neurons stimulate gastrin secretion directly (via M_3 receptors) as well as indirectly by inhibiting SST secretion (via M_2 and M_4 receptors). GRP neurons, activated by luminal protein, stimulate gastrin secretion directly. VIP neurons, activated by low-grade distension, stimulate SST (via VPAC-1 receptors) and thus inhibit gastrin secretion. PACAP neurons, acting via PAC-1 receptors, stimulate histamine secretion and, acting via VPAC-1 receptors, stimulate SST secretion; the net effect of PACAP on acid secretion will depend upon the relative contribution of these pathways. Dual paracrine pathways link SST-containing D cells to parietal and ECL cells in the fundus/body. Histamine released from ECL cells acts via H_3 receptors to inhibit SST secretion; this pathway serves to accentuate the decrease in SST secretion induced by cholinergic stimuli and thus augments acid secretion. In the antrum, dual paracrine pathways link SST and gastrin secretion. Release of acid into the lumen of the stomach restores SST secretion in both the fundus/body and antrum; the latter is mediated by release of CGRP from extrinsic sensory neurons.

Histamine

Histamine is produced in ECL cells located at the base of oxyntic glands. These cells possess neural-like cytoplasmic processes that terminate in the vicinity of parietal cells [23]. Histamine receptors have been classified into four major subclasses: H_1, H_2, H_3, and H_4. The H_4 receptor shares 40% homology and over-lapping pharmacology with the H_3 receptor. Histamine is thought to be the most important direct activator of the parietal cell. It stimulates the parietal cell by binding to H_2 receptors on its basolateral membrane that activate AC to generate adenosine that, in turn, generates adenosine 3′,5′-cyclic monophosphate (cAMP)

[24]. Cyclic AMP activates cAMP-dependent protein kinase (protein kinase A (PKA)) that phosphorylates various intracellular proteins (e.g., the actin binding proteins, ezrin and lasp-1), resulting in acid secretion [25] (Figure 5.2). *In vitro* studies of H_3 agonists and antagonists suggest that local release of histamine in the stomach also may stimulate acid secretion indirectly by binding to H_3 receptors that inhibit SST release [26, 27] (Figure 5.3).

Gastrin

Gastrin, the main stimulant of acid secretion during a meal, is released in response to dietary proteins, amino acids, and amines as well as by gastric distension [28–31]. Gastrin is produced in G cells of the gastric antrum and, in much lower amounts, in the proximal small intestine, colon, and pancreas [32]. The major stored form of gastrin in the antrum is G17, whereas the duodenum contains equal amounts of G17 and G34. Because the plasma half-life of G17 is 3–7 min but that of G34 is 30 min, most gastrin in the circulation during fasting is G34. Both forms are metabolized primarily by the kidney but also by the intestine [33]. Thus, serum gastrin may be elevated in patients with renal insufficiency and massive small bowel resection. The upper limit of normal fasting gastrin concentration is approximately 100 pg/ml (~50 pmol/l); in response to a meal, this concentration increases to approximately 300 pg/ml (~150 pmol/l).

Gastrin and Gastrin and cholecystokinin (CCK) belong to the same peptide family and possess an identical carboxyl-terminal pentapeptide sequence. Two main classes of gastrin and CCK receptors have been characterized: CCK_1 (formerly CCK-A (alimentary)) and CCK_2 (formerly CCK-B (brain) or CCK-B/gastrin). Gastrin acts via CCK_2 receptors to stimulate the parietal cell directly and, more importantly, indirectly by releasing histamine from ECL cells [34, 35] (Figure 5.2 and Figure 5.3). H_2 receptor-deficient mice do not produce acid in response to histamine or gastrin [36].

A variety of factors regulate gastrin expression and secretion, including neuropeptides, inflammatory cytokines, meal-related nutrients, and luminal pH. ACh, GRP, protein, amino acids, amines, calcium, and alcoholic beverages produced by fermentation stimulate, whereas SST and interleukin-1β inhibit gastrin secretion [29, 37, 38]. The calcium-sensing receptor and the L-amino acid receptor (GPRC6A) have been identified on G cells and may provide a mechanism by which G cells directly sense luminal proteins and their breakdown products [39]. In addition, two negative feedback pathways, mediated through release of SST, regulate gastrin secretion. The first is activated by luminal acidity and involves sensory CGRP neurons (Figure 5.3). Low intragastric pH (high intragastric acidity) activates CGRP neurons that stimulate SST and thus inhibit gastrin secretion [40, 41]. Conversely, when intragastric pH rises (low intragastric acidity), for example, due to the effects of gastric atrophy or antisecretory drugs such as proton pump inhibitors (PPIs), SST secretion is inhibited and gastrin stimulated, resulting in hypergastrinemia. The second feedback pathway involves a paracrine pathway whereby gastrin directly stimulates SST and thus attenuates its own secretion [42].

Gastrin, acting through CCK_2 receptors, also functions as a trophic hormone that stimulates proliferation of gastric mucosal cells, including parietal and ECL cells. Accordingly, chronic hypergastrinemia, due to either a gastrin-producing tumor or antisecretory medications, induces proliferation of parietal and ECL cells [43]. In Zollinger–Ellison syndrome (ZES), an acid hypersecretory disorder caused by a gastrin-producing tumor (gastrinoma), hypergastrinemia produces rugal hypertrophy. After 2 months of PPI treatment, resultant hypergastrinemia induces parietal and ECL hyperplasia that persists for 2–3 months after stopping the PPI [44]. The clinical consequence is rebound acid secretion, which may exacerbate gastroesophageal reflux disease, induce dyspeptic symptoms, and provoke symptoms in patients with duodenal ulcer disease [45].

Acetylcholine
In oxyntic mucosa, ACh released from postganglionic neurons whose cell bodies are located primarily in the submucosal plexus stimulates the parietal cell directly via M_3 receptors that increase intracellular calcium and trisphosphate concentrations (Figure 5.2) and indirectly by inhibiting SST secretion via M_2 and M_4 receptors [46] (Figure 5.3). Inhibition of SST secretion removes the tonic restraint exerted by this peptide on ECL and parietal cells [47, 48]. ACh does not appear to stimulate histamine secretion from ECL cells [49, 50]. In pyloric mucosa, ACh stimulates gastrin secretion directly via M_3 receptors on G cells and indirectly via M_2 and M_4 receptors on D cells coupled to inhibition of SST secretion [51, 52] (Figure 5.3).

Gastrin-releasing peptide
GRP immunoreactivity has been identified in gastric mucosal neurons and GRP receptors have been identified on gastrin-containing G cells [53]. Endogenous GRP, released in response to luminal protein, stimulates gastrin secretion [29] (Figure 5.3).

Pituitary adenylate cyclase-activating polypeptide
PACAP, a member of the secretin–glucagon–VIP family of peptides, is present in gastric intramural neurons [54]. Its effects are mediated via three distinct receptors: PACAP receptor type-1 (PAC-1), VPAC-1 (the classic VIP receptor), and VPAC-2. The PAC-1 receptor has high affinity for PACAP but low affinity for VIP, whereas VPAC-1 and VPAC-2 receptors have near-equal affinity for PACAP and VIP [55]. In the stomach, PAC-1 receptors have been identified on histamine-containing ECL cells and VPAC-1 receptors on SST-containing D cells [56]. Exogenous PACAP has been reported to either stimulate or inhibit acid secretion, depending upon the relative contribution of histamine release from ECL cells and SST release from D cells [57, 58]. In rat, a PACAP receptor antagonist attenuates acid secretion, implying that endogenous PACAP stimulates acid secretion [58].

Somatostatin

SST is the main inhibitor of gastric acid secretion. Its actions are mediated via five G-protein coupled receptors (GPCRs), named SSTR1–SSTR5. SSTR2, the predominant receptor regulating gastric acid secretion, is present on ECL, parietal, and gastrin cells [59–61] (Figure 5.2 and Figure 5.3). In the stomach, SST cells are coupled to their target cells by cytoplasmic processes [14] that release SST, which exerts a tonic paracrine restraint on ECL cell histamine secretion, parietal cell acid secretion, and G-cell gastrin secretion [62, 63] (Figure 5.2 and 5.3). Removal of this restraint (i.e., disinhibition) by activation of cholinergic neurons is an important physiologic mechanism for stimulating acid secretion. As mentioned in the section "Gastrin", an increase in luminal acidity acts to attenuate acid secretion via a pathway involving release of SST in the fundus, corpus, and antrum [64].

Enterogastrone

An enterogastrone is an intestinal factor that inhibits gastric acid secretion when nutrients are present in the intestine. Prime candidates include CCK, secretin, neurotensin, gastric inhibitory peptide, glucagon-like peptide, glicentin, and oxyntomodulin. All are found in intestinal mucosa, released into the circulation in response to luminal lipids and carbohydrates, and capable of inhibiting acid secretion at physiologically relevant blood concentrations [65, 66]. Although enterogastrone activity likely represents the combined influence of several of these peptides, the strongest evidence favors CCK, which is released from I cells in the proximal intestine by luminal lipid and protein. The acid inhibitory effect of CCK is primarily mediated by activation of CCK_1 receptors coupled to release of gastric SST [67, 68].

Parietal cell intracellular pathways

Acid secretion from parietal cells is accomplished by activation of intracellular cAMP and calcium-dependent signaling pathways. These activate downstream protein kinases, ultimately leading to fusion and activation of the proton pump of the parietal cell, hydrogen–potassium-stimulated adenosine triphosphatase (H^+K^+-ATPase), with concomitant activation of luminal membrane K^+ and Cl^- conductance [10, 69] (Figure 5.4). H^+K^+-ATPase actively pumps H^+ out of the cell in exchange for K^+. Cl^- is secreted concurrently into the lumen through apical Cl^- channels to create hydrochloric acid. Putative Cl^- channels include chloride intracellular channel-6 (CLIC-6), cystic fibrosis transmembrane regulator (CFTR), and SLC26A9 [70, 71]. Cl^- is loaded into the cell via the basolateral Cl^-/HCO_3^- anion exchanger (AE2 or SLC4A2), the sodium-2–chloride–potassium cotransporter (NKCCl), and the SLC26A7 Cl^- channel [69]. A molecule of HCO_3^- exits the cells across the basolateral membrane for each H^+ secreted. Entry of HCO_3^- from parietal cells into blood has been referred to as the "alkaline tide." Some of this HCO_3^- is taken up and secreted by surface epithelial cells.

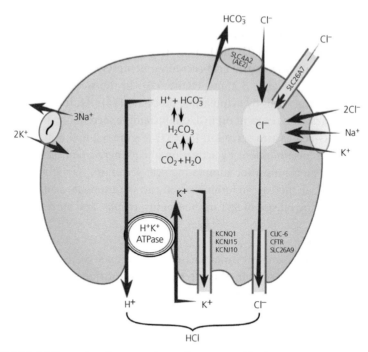

Figure 5.4 Model illustrating the generation and secretion of hydrochloric acid (HCl) by the parietal cell. Acid secretion requires a functional H^+K^+-ATPase as well as apical K^+ (KCNQ1, KCNJ15, and/or KCNJ10) and Cl^- (CFTR, CLIC-6, and/or CLC26A9) channels and basolateral Cl^- channels (SLC26A7), exchangers (Cl^-/HCO_3^- anion exchanger 2 (AE2 or SLC4A2)), and transporters (NKCCl or Na^+-2Cl^-K^+ cotransporter). Acid is produced by the hydration of CO_2 to form $H^+ + HCO_3^-$, a reaction catalyzed by cytoplasmic carbonic anhydrase CA. For each H^+ secreted, a HCO_3^- exits the cell via the basolateral AE2.

H^+K^+-ATPase is composed of an α-subunit that contains the catalytic site and is responsible for actual ion exchange and a β-subunit that protects the enzyme from degradation and is necessary for trafficking to and from the luminal membrane. In the resting state, H^+K^+-ATPase is sequestered within cytoplasmic tubulovesicles and is inactive. During stimulation, the enzyme is translocated into the apical membrane and becomes active. The precise pathways regulating membrane translocation and fusion are not known [72].

Measurement of gastric acid secretion

Gastric secretory testing measures the basal and maximal capacity of the stomach to produce acid. It no longer has much clinical utility, but may assist in the diagnosis and management of patients with hypergastrinemia (e.g., ZES) and in the diagnosis of incomplete vagotomy in patients with postoperative ulcer recurrence. Normal acid secretion or a fasting acidic gastric pH excludes the diagnosis of achlorhydria as the cause of an elevated fasting serum gastrin concentration. Gastrinoma patients exhibit hypergastrinemia with elevated basal acid output (BAO).

The most widely used method for measuring gastric acid secretion is aspiration of gastric juice through a nasogastric tube positioned in the most dependent portion of the stomach during fasting. An endoscopic technique recently has been described whereby all gastric contents are aspirated and discarded and then a single 15-min sample of juice is collected under direct endoscopic observation [73].

The H^+ concentration in a sample of gastric juice can be determined by back-titration with sodium hydroxide. The millimoles (mmol) of base needed to titrate a volume of gastric juice to pH 7 represent the "titratable" acidity in mmol per liter of sample. The H^+ concentration of the sample in mmol per liter is then multiplied by the volume of the sample in liters to determine the acid output during the collection period (e.g., mmol per hour or mmol per kilogram of body weight per hour).

BAO estimates resting acid secretion and is expressed as the sum of the measured acid output, in mmol H^+ per hour, for four consecutive 15-min periods. The upper limit of normal for men and women is 10 and 8 mmol/h, respectively. BAO varies during the day, with the lowest rates occurring in the early morning before breakfast and the highest rates occurring in the evening. Variation is also related to cyclic gastric motor activity, with increased BAO in late gastric phase III of the migrating motor complex [74].

Maximal acid output (MAO) and peak acid output (PAO) estimate the acid secretory response to an exogenous secretagogue, usually pentagastrin. MAO is the sum of acid output of four consecutive 15-min collection periods, and PAO, which correlates with parietal cell mass (i.e., the number of functional parietal cells), is calculated by multiplying the sum of the two highest outputs recorded in the four test periods by two. Normal MAO levels range from 10 to 50 mmol/h for men and 5 to 30 mmol/h for women. PAO is somewhat higher than MAO and ranges from 10 to 60 mmol H^+/h. BAO averages about 10% of MAO and rarely exceeds 20%.

Regulation of pepsinogen secretion

Pepsinogens are inactive proenzymes, termed zymogens, that are synthesized primarily in chief cells but also in mucous neck cells. Pepsinogens are converted to pepsins by luminal gastric acid. Pepsins are optimally active at pH 1.8–3.5, reversibly inactivated at pH 5, and irreversibly denatured at pH 7. Pepsins act in concert with acid to digest dietary proteins and may also be important for killing ingested bacteria [75].

Group I pepsinogens (PGI; old term, pepsinogen A) are expressed in chief and mucous cells of the oxyntic mucosa. Group II pepsinogens (PGII; old term, pepsinogen C), which represent 20% of total pepsin content, are expressed in oxyntic and pyloric mucosa as well as in duodenal Brunner's glands [76]. ACh released from intramural cholinergic neurons is the most important physiologic stimulant for pepsinogen secretion. Other stimulants include gastrin, histamine, CCK, and GRP.

Serum levels of PGI correlate with acid output. A linear relationship exists between the loss of chief cells in patients with oxyntic atrophy and serum PGI levels; a PGI concentration less than $30\,\mu g/L$ or PGI to PGII ratio of 2.5–3.0 or less has been used as a noninvasive test to detect atrophic gastritis [77]. It should be noted that PGI is increased in the serum of humans treated with PPIs, although the precise mechanism for this increase is unknown [78]. Serum PGII concentration is elevated in *Helicobacter pylori* infection and a decrease of 23% or greater recently has been reported to detect successful eradication with 100% sensitivity and 97% specificity [79].

Gastric defense

A number of premucosal, mucosal, and submucosal defense mechanisms protect the gastric mucosa from acid-peptic injury [80, 81] (Figure 5.5). Premucosal gastric defense consists of a physical barrier of bicarbonate and mucin secreted by the gastric epithelium. If the buffering capacity of this barrier were absent, the gastric surface pH would approach that of the lumen. Bicarbonate, however, is actively secreted by parietal and surface epithelial cells to create a gradient such that the epithelium is exposed to a pH of 4.0–7.0 when the gastric luminal pH is as low as 2.0. The production of bicarbonate is primarily mediated by prostaglandins, specifically prostaglandin E_2 (PGE2) [83]. Prostaglandins are made from arachidonic acid by the cyclooxygenases (COXs), cyclooxygenase-1 (COX-1) and cyclooxygenase-2 (COX-2). Inhibitors of COX-1, such as nonsteroidal anti-inflammatory drugs (NSAIDs), potentiate gastric mucosal injury, in part by decreasing bicarbonate secretion. Prostaglandin E synthase, the enzyme responsible for catalyzing conversion of PGH2 to PGE2, is upregulated in response to gastric mucosal damage and accelerates ulcer healing through stimulation of bicarbonate, mucous, and phospholipid secretion. PGE2 also increases blood flow and mucosal repair [84].

The phospholipid caps and tight junctions of gastric epithelial cells act as physical barriers to injury and prevent back diffusion of acid into the subepithelial space (Figure 5.5). Trefoil-factor family peptides, secreted with mucins, increase mucous-layer viscosity and promote mucosal restitution independent of COX-mediated prostaglandin synthesis [85, 86]. Growth factors (e.g., basic fibroblast growth factor, hypoxia-inducible factor, and vascular endothelial growth factor) promote healing by increasing angiogenesis [87, 88]. Heme oxygenase-1, a stress-inducible reactive oxygen species-scavenging enzyme, protects against

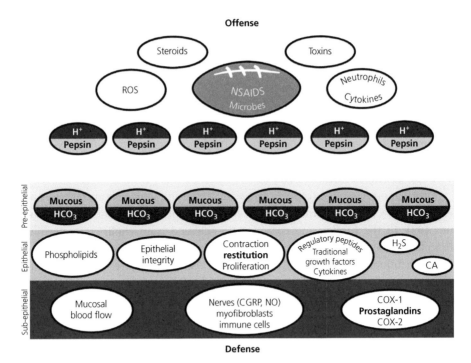

Figure 5.5 Gastroduodenal offense and defense. Mucosal integrity depends upon a delicate balance between aggressive and defensive factors. When mucosal defense mechanisms are overwhelmed, ulceration may occur. NSAIDs, nonsteroidal anti-inflammatory drugs; ROS, reactive oxygen species; HCO_3, bicarbonate; H_2S, hydrogen sulfide; CA, carbonic anhydrase; CGRP, calcitonin gene-related peptide; NO, nitric oxide; COX-1, cyclooxygenase-1; COX-2, cyclooxygenase-2. From Reference [82]. Reproduced with permission of Elsevier.

NSAID-induced gastric injury as does NO and hydrogen sulfide (H_2S) [89]. Carbonic anhydrase (CA) generates HCO_3^- from CO_2 and H_2O (Figure 5.4 and Figure 5.5).

The submucosal microcirculation supplies the mucosa with oxygen, bicarbonate, and nutrients while removing toxins and acid. It is also important in removing bicarbonate produced on the basolateral membrane of the parietal cell during acid production. This "alkaline tide" is absorbed by the local circulation and distributed to surface epithelial cells where it is taken up by sodium bicarbonate cotransporters and then secreted to provide the protective pre-epithelial alkaline layer [90]. A number of neurotransmitters protect the gastric mucosa including CGRP, NO, and H_2S. CGRP, a neurotransmitter, protects the mucosa against damage through its vasodilatory, anti-inflammatory, antiapoptotic, and antioxidant effects, some of which are mediated by release of NO [91, 92]. H_2S upregulates gastric mucosal blood flow, inhibits leukocyte–endothelial cell adhesion, and serves as an antioxidant [93].

Physiologic correlates

Response to a meal

Gastric intramural neurons are the primary regulators of acid secretion. These effector neurons act on parietal cells directly and also indirectly by regulating the secretion of SST, gastrin, and possibly histamine (Figure 5.3). In the basal state, acid secretion is maintained at a low level by the tonic restraint of SST on ECL (histamine) and parietal (acid) cells in the fundus and corpus and on G (gastrin) cells in the antrum. Cholinergic neural stimulation removes SST inhibition and promotes gastrin and acid secretion.

Anticipation of a meal (cephalic phase of digestion) activates central neurons whose input is relayed by the vagus nerve to gastric intramural cholinergic neurons [94]. In the fundus and corpus, ACh released from cholinergic neurons stimulates parietal cells directly and also indirectly by eliminating the inhibitory paracrine influence of SST on ECL and parietal cells [95] (Figure 5.3). The resulting increase in histamine stimulates the parietal cell directly via H_2 receptors and indirectly via H_3 receptors [26, 96]. Histamine, acting on H_3 receptors, amplifies the ability of secretagogues to stimulate acid secretion by further suppressing SST secretion. Thus, the net effect of cholinergic neural stimulation is suppression of paracrine inhibitory influences (i.e., SST) and enhancement of stimulatory influences (i.e., ACh and histamine).

In the antrum, cholinergic neurons activated by anticipation of a meal stimulate gastrin secretion directly as well as indirectly by suppressing SST secretion (Figure 5.3). Gastrin, in turn, stimulates the parietal cell directly and, more importantly, indirectly by enhancing secretion of histamine [97] (Figure 5.2 and Figure 5.3).

As food enters the stomach, the same cholinergic neurons are further activated mechanically by distension and chemically by protein [28–31]. Initially, the meal buffers secreted acid. There is activation of CGRP neurons and a further decrease in SST secretion and thus increase in gastrin secretion. The decrease in acidity leads to decreased activation of CGRP neurons resulting in a further decrease in somatostatin and thus increase in gastrin secretion [29, 98]. It is worth emphasizing that suppression of SST secretion permits an optimal gastrin response.

As food leaves the stomach, pathways are activated that restore the inhibitory influence of SST. First, a stimulatory paracrine pathway linking gastrin to antral SST cells is activated to restore antral SST secretion after gastrin release [42] (Figure 5.3). Second, there is decreased activation of cholinergic neurons by anticipation of the meal, distension, and protein. Third, as distension decreases, VIP neurons that stimulate SST secretion are preferentially activated [28]. Fourth, as the buffering capacity of the meal is lost, luminal acidification stimulates SST secretion. Fifth, enterogastrones released from the small intestine in response to nutrients (e.g., CCK and secretin) stimulate SST secretion [65]. The resultant increase in gastric SST secretion attenuates gastrin and acid secretion, thus restoring the basal state. This state is manifest by the continuous restraint exerted on parietal (acid), ECL (histamine), and G (gastrin) cells by contiguous SST cells. A decrease in this restraint is sufficient to again initiate acid secretion.

Acknowledgment

The author thanks Mary Beatty-Brooks for the artwork.

Multiple choice questions

1 During the interdigestive period, gastric acid secretion is maintained at an economically low level primarily by the action of:
   A Histamine released from oxyntic enterochromaffin-like cells
   B Gastrin released from pyloric G cells
   C Acetylcholine released from postganglionic intramural neurons
   D Somatostatin released from oxyntic and pyloric D cells
2 The following factors or disorders lead to increased gastrin secretion:
   A Somatostatin, luminal proteins, and increased luminal acidity
   B Zollinger–Ellison syndrome, acetylcholine, and secretin
   C High distension, luminal proteins, and decreased luminal acidity
   D Cholecystokinin, histamine, and increased luminal acidity
3 A 75-year-old woman presents with osteopenia and hip fracture. She is not taking proton pump inhibitors. Laboratory findings that would best assist in diagnosing the underlying disorder would be the following:
   A Normal serum gastrin and normal serum pepsinogen I
   B Hypergastrinemia with low serum levels of pepsinogen I
   C Hypergastrinemia and high normal basal acid output
   D Elevated pepsinogen II and elevated serum iron
4 *One best answer*: All the following factors contribute to the mucosal barrier (which protect the stomach from self-digestion) except:
   A Endogenous prostaglandins
   B Maintenance of the submucosal circulation
   C Endogenous corticoids
   D The mucus coat, containing trapped HCO_3
   E Nitric oxide

References

1 Hutchinson, C., Geissler, C.A., Powell, J.J. and Bomford, A. (2007) Proton pump inhibitors suppress absorption of dietary non-haem iron in hereditary haemochromatosis. *Gut* , **56**, 1291–1295.
2 O'Connell, M.B., Madden, D.M., Murray, A.M. *et al.* (2005) Effects of proton pump inhibitors on calcium carbonate absorption in women: a randomized crossover trial. *American Journal of Medicine*, **118**, 778–781.

3 Gray, S.L., LaCroix, A.Z., Larson, J. *et al.* (2010) Proton pump inhibitor use, hip fracture, and change in bone mineral density in postmenopausal women: results from the women's health initiative. *Archives of Internal Medicine*, **170**, 765–771.

4 Den Elzen, W.P.J., Groeneveld, Y., De Ruijter, W. *et al.* (2008) Long-term use of proton pump inhibitors and vitamin B12 status in elderly individuals. *Alimentary Pharmacology Therapeutics*, **27**, 491–497.

5 Lahner, E., Annibale, B. and Delle Fave, G. (2009) Systematic review: impaired drug absorption related to the co-administration of antisecretory therapy. *Alimentary Pharmacology Therapeutics*, **12**, 1219–1229.

6 Lombardo, L., Foti, M., Ruggia, O. and Chiecchio, A. (2010) Increased incidence of small intestinal bacterial overgrowth during proton pump inhibitor therapy. *Clinical Gastroenterology and Hepatology*, **8**, 504–508.

7 Bajaj, J.S., Zadvornova, Y., Heuman, D.M. *et al.* (2009) Association of proton pump inhibitor therapy with spontaneous bacterial peritonitis in cirrhotic patients with ascites. *The American Journal of Gastroenterology*, **104**, 1130–1134.

8 Janarthanan, S., Ditah, I., Phil, M. *et al.* (2012) *Clostridium difficile*-associated diarrhea and proton pump inhibitor therapy: a meta-analysis. *The American Journal of Gastroenterology*, **107**, 1001–1010.

9 Pali-Scholl, I. and Jensen-Jarolim, E. (2011) Anti-acid medication as a risk factor for food allergy. *Allergy*, **66**, 469–477.

10 Schubert, M.L. (2012) Regulation of gastric acid secretion, in *Physiology of the Gastrointestinal Tract*, 5th edn (ed. L.R. Johnson), Academic Press, Oxford. pp. 1281–1310.

11 Chandrasoma, P. (2005) Controversies of the cardiac mucosa and Barrett's oesophagus. *Histopathology*, **46**, 361–373.

12 Hirsch, A.B., McCuen, R.W., Arimura, A. and Schubert, M.L. (2003) Adrenomedullin stimulates somatostatin and thus inhibits histamine and acid secretion in the fundus of the stomach. *Regulatory Peptides*, **110**, 189–195.

13 Zaki, M., Koduru, S., McCuen, R. *et al.* (2012) Amylin, released from the gastric fundus, stimulates somatostatin and thus inhibits histamine and acid secretion in mice. *Gastroenterology*, **123**, 247–255.

14 Larsson, L-I., Goltermann, N., DeMagistris, L. *et al.* (1979) Somatostatin cell processes as pathways for paracrine secretion. *Science*, **205**, 1393–1395.

15 Zhao, C.M., Furnes, M.W., Stenstrom, B. *et al.* (2008) Characterization of obestatin- and ghrelin-producing cells in the gastrointestinal tract and pancreas of rats: an immunohistochemical and electron-microscopic study. *Cell and Tissue Research*, **331**, 575–587.

16 Chen, D., Zhao, C.M., Lindström, E. and Håkanson, R. (1999) Rat stomach ECL cells – update of biology and physiology. *General Pharmacology*, **32**, 413–422.

17 Schubert, M.L., Edwards, N.F., Arimura, A. and Makhlouf, G.M. (1987) Paracrine regulation of gastric acid secretion by fundic somatostatin. *American Journal of Physiology – Gastrointestinal and Liver Physiology*, **252**, G485–G490.

18 Saffouri, B., Weir, G.C., Bitar, K.N. and Makhlouf, G.M. (1979) Stimulation of gastrin secretion from the perfused rat stomach by somatostatin antiserum. *Life Sciences*, **25**, 1749–1754.

19 Gower, W.R., Jr., Premaratne, S., McCuen, R.W. *et al.* (2003) Gastric atrial natriuretic peptide regulates endocrine secretion in antrum and fundus of human and rat stomach. *American Journal of Physiology – Gastrointestinal and Liver Physiology*, **284**, G638–G645.

20 Yu, P.L., Fujimura, M., Hayashi, N. *et al.* (2001) Mechanisms in regulating the release of serotonin from the perfused rat stomach. *American Journal of Physiology – Gastrointestinal and Liver Physiology*, **280**, G1099–G1105.

21 De la Cour, C.D., Björkqvist, M., Sandvik, A.K. *et al.* (2001) A-like cells in the rat stomach contain ghrelin and do not operate under gastrin control. *Regulatory Peptides*, **99**, 141–150.

22 Furness, J.B. (2000) Types of neurons in the enteric nervous system. *Journal of the Autonomic Nervous System*, **81**, 87–96.

23 Gustafsson, B.I., Bakke, I., Hauso, O. *et al.* (2011) Parietal cell activation by arborization of ECL cell cytoplasmic projections is likely the mechanism of histamine induced secretion of hydrochloric acid. *Scandinavian Journal of Gastroenterology*, **46**, 531–537.

24 Chew, C.S. (1985) Parietal cell protein kinases. Selective activation of type 1 cAMP-dependent protein kinase by histamine. *The Journal of Biological Chemistry*, **260**, 7540–7550.

25 Tamura, A., Kikuchi, S., Hata, M. *et al.* (2005) Achlorhydria by ezrin knockdown: defects in the formation/expansion of apical canaliculi in gastric parietal cells. *The Journal of Cell Biology*, **169**, 21–28.

26 Vuyyuru, L., Schubert, M.L., Harrington, L. *et al.* (1995) Dual inhibitory pathways link antral somatostatin and histamine secretion in human, dog, and rat stomach. *Gastroenterology*, **109**, 1566–1574.

27 Bado, A., Moizo, L., Laigneau, J.P. *et al.* (1994) H_3-receptor regulation of vascular gastrin and somatostatin releases by the isolated rat stomach. *Yale Journal of Biology and Medicine*, **67**, 113–121.

28 Schubert, M.L. and Makhlouf, G.M. (1993) Gastrin secretion induced by distension is regulated by cholinergic and vasoactive intestinal peptide neurons in rats. *Gastroenterology*, **104**, 834–839.

29 Schubert, M.L., Coy, D.H. and Makhlouf, G.M. (1992) Peptone stimulates gastrin secretion from the stomach by activating bombesin/GRP and cholinergic neurons. *American Journal of Physiology – Gastrointestinal and Liver Physiology*, **262**, G685–G689.

30 Schiller, L.R., Walsh, J.H. and Feldman, M. (1980) Distension-induced gastrin release. *Gastroenterology*, **78**, 912–917.

31 Lichtenberger, L.M., Delansorne, R. and Graziani, L.A. (1982) Importance of amino acid uptake and decarboxylation in gastrin release from isolated G cells. *Nature London*, **295**, 698–700.

32 Dockray, G.J., Varro, A., Dimaline, R. and Wang, T. (2001) The gastrins: their production and biological activities. *Annual Review of Physiology*, **63**, 119–139.

33 Hansen, C.P., Stadil, F., Yucun, L. and Rehfeld, J.F. (1996) Pharmacokinetics and organ metabolism of carboxyamidated and glycine-extended gastrins in pigs. *American Journal of Physiology – Gastrointestinal and Liver Physiology*, **271**, G156–G163.

34 Waldum, H.L., Sandvik, A.K., Brenna, E. and Petersen, H. (1991) Gastrin-histamine sequence in the regulation of gastric acid secretion. *Gut*, **32**, 698–701.

35 Schubert, M.L. and Peura, D.A. (2008) Control of gastric acid secretion in health and disease. *Gastroenterology*, **134**, 1842–1860.

36 Kobayashi, T., Tonai, S., Ishihara, Y. *et al.* (2000) Abnormal functional and morphological regulation of the gastric mucosa in histamine H2 receptor-deficient mice. *Journal of Clinical Investigation*, **105**, 1741–1749.

37 Ericsson, P., Hakanson, R. and Norlen, P. (2010) Gastrin response to candidate messengers in intact conscious rats monitored by antrum microdialysis. *Regulatory Peptides*, **163**, 24–30.

38 Kidd, M., Hauso, O., Drozdov, I. *et al.* (2009) Delineation of the chemomechanosensory regulation of gastrin secretion using pure rodent G cells. *Gastroenterology*, **137**, 231–241.

39 Feng, J., Petersen, C.D., Coy, D.H. *et al.* (2010) Calcium-sensing receptor is a physiologic multimodal chemosensor regulating gastric G-cell growth and gastrin secretion. *Proceedings of the National Academy of Science USA*, **107**, 17791–17796.

40 Brand, S. and Stone, D. (1988) Reciprocal regulation of antral gastrin and somatostatin gene expression by omeprazole-induced achlorhydria. *Journal of Clinical Investigation*, **82**, 1059–1066.

41 Manela, F.D., Ren, J., Gao, J. *et al.* (1995) Calcitonin gene-related peptide modulates acid-mediated regulation of somatostatin and gastrin release from rat antrum. *Gastroenterology*, **109**, 701–706.

42 Schubert, M.L., Jong, M.J. and Makhlouf, G.M. (1991) Bombesin/GRP-stimulated somatostatin secretion is mediated by gastrin in the antrum and intrinsic neurons in the fundus. *American Journal of Physiology – Gastrointestinal and Liver Physiology*, **261**, G885–G889.

43 Ryberg, B., Tielemans, Y., Axelson, J. *et al.* (1990) Gastrin stimulates the self-replication rate of enterochromaffinlike cells in the rat stomach. Effects of omeprazole, ranitidine, and gastrin-17 in intact and antrectomized rats. *Gastroenterology*, **99**, 935–942.

44 Waldum, H.L., Qvigstad, G., Fossmark, R. *et al.* (2010) Rebound acid hypersecretion from a physiological, pathophysiological and clinical viewpoint. *Scandinavian Journal of Gastroenterology*, **45**, 389–394.

45 Reimer, C., Sondergaard, B., Hilsted, L. and Bytzer, P. (2009) Proton-pump inhibitor therapy induces acid-related symptoms in healthy volunteers after withdrawal of therapy. *Gastroenterology*, **137**, 80–87.

46 Leonard, A., Cuq, P., Magous, R. and Bali, J.-P. (1991) M3-subtype muscarinic receptor that controls intracellular calcium release and inositol phosphate accumulation in gastric parietal cells. *Biochemical Pharmacology*, **42**, 839–845.

47 Schubert, M.L., Saffouri, B. and Makhlouf, G.M. (1988) Identical patterns of somatostatin secretion from isolated antrum and fundus of rat stomach. *American Journal of Physiology – Gastrointestinal and Liver Physiology*, **254**, G20–G24.

48 Schubert, M.L. and Hightower, J. (1990) Functionally distinct muscarinic receptors on gastric somatostatin cells. *American Journal of Physiology – Gastrointestinal and Liver Physiology*, **258**, G982–G987.

49 Lindström, E. and Håkanson, R. (2001) Neurohormonal regulation of secretion from isolated rat stomach ECL cells: a critical reappraisal. *Regulatory Peptides*, **97**, 169–180.

50 Athmann, C., Zeng, N.X., Scott, D.R. and Sachs, G. (2000) Regulation of parietal cell calcium signaling in gastric glands. *American Journal of Physiology – Gastrointestinal and Liver Physiology*, **279**, G1048–G1058.

51 Yokotani, K., DelValle, J., Park, J. and Yamada, T. (1995) Muscarinic M_3 receptor-mediated release of gastrin from canine antral G cells in primary culture. *Digestion*, **56**, 31–34.

52 Koop, I., Squires, P.E., Meloche, R.M. *et al.* (1997) Effect of cholinergic agonists on gastrin release from primary cultures of human antral G cells. *Gastroenterology*, **112**, 357–363.

53 Baldwin, G.S., Patel, O. and Sulkes, A. (2007) Phylogenetic analysis of the sequences of gastrin-releasing peptide and its receptors: biological implications. *Regulatory Peptides*, **143**, 1–14.

54 Miampamba, M., Germano, P.M., Arli, S. *et al.* (2002) Expression of pituitary adenylate cyclase-activating polypeptide and PACAP type 1 receptor in the rat gastric and colonic myenteric neurons. *Regulatory Peptides*, **105**, 145–154.

55 Pisegna, J.R. and Oh, D.S.(2007) Pituitary adenylate cyclase-activating polypeptide: a novel peptide with protean implications. *Current Opinion in Endocrinology, Diabetes and Obesity*, **14**, 58–62.

56 Zeng, N.X., Kang, T., Lyu, R.M. *et al.* (1998) The pituitary adenylate cyclase activating polypeptide type 1 receptor (PAC_1-R) is expressed on gastric ECL cells: evidence by immunocytochemistry and RT-PCR. *Annals of the New York Academy of Sciences*, **865**, 147–156.

57 Piqueras, L., Taché, Y. and Martínez, V. (2004) Peripheral PACAP inhibits gastric acid secretion through somatostatin release in mice. *British Journal of Pharmacology*, **142**:67–78.

58 Sandvik, A.K., Cui, G.L., Bakke, I. *et al.* (2001) PACAP stimulates gastric acid secretion in the rat by inducing histamine release. *American Journal of Physiology – Gastrointestinal and Liver Physiology*, **281**, G997–G1003.

59 Allen, J.P., Canty, A.J., Schulz, S. *et al.* (2002) Identification of cells expressing somatostatin receptor 2 in the gastrointestinal tract of *Sstr2* knockout/*lacZ* knockin mice. *Journal of Comparative Neurology*, **454**, 329–340.

60 Zaki, M., Harrington, L., McCuen, R. *et al.* (1996) Somatostatin receptor subtype 2 mediates inhibition of gastrin and histamine secretion from human, dog, and rat antrum. *Gastroenterology*, **111**, 919–924.

61 Prinz, C., Sachs, G., Walsh, J.H. *et al.* (1994) The somatostatin receptor subtype on rat enterochromaffinlike cells. *Gastroenterology*, **107**, 1067–1074.

62 Makhlouf, G.M. and Schubert, M.L. (1990) Gastric somatostatin: a paracrine regulator of acid secretion. *Metabolism*, **39** (Suppl 2), 138–142.

63 Short, G.M., Doyle, W. and Wolfe, M.M. (1985) Effect of antibodies to somatostatin on acid secretion and gastrin release by isolated perfused rat stomach. *Gastroenterology*, **88**, 984–988.

64 Schubert, M.L., Edwards, N.F. and Makhlouf, G.M. (1988) Regulation of gastric somatostatin secretion in the mouse by luminal acid: a local feedback mechanism. *Gastroenterology*, **94**, 317–322.

65 Schubert, M.L. (2008) Hormonal regulation of gastric acid secretion. *Current Gastroenterology Reports*, **10**, 523–527.

66 Holst, J.J. (2007) The physiology of glucagon-like peptide 1. *Physiological Reviews*, **87**, 1409–1439.

67 Lloyd, K.C.K., Maxwell, V., Chuang, C-N. *et al.* (1994) Somatostatin is released in response to cholecystokinin by activation of type A CCK receptors. *Peptides*, **15**, 223–227.

68 Whited, K.L., Thao, D., Lloyd, K.C.K. *et al.* (2006) Targeted disruption of the murine CCK1 receptor gene reduces intestinal lipid-induced feedback inhibition of gastric function. *American Journal of Physiology – Gastrointestinal and Liver Physiology*, **291**, G156–G162.

69 Kopic, S. and Geibel, J.P. (2010) Update on the mechanisms of gastric acid secretion. *Current Gastroenterology Reports*, **12**, 458–464.

70 Sidani, S.M., Kirchhoff, P., Socrates, T. *et al.* (2007) Delta F508 mutation results in impaired gastric acid secretion. *Journal of Biological Chemistry*, **282**, 6068–6074.

71 Xu, J., Henriksnäs, J., Barone, S. *et al.* (2005 Aug) SLC26A9 is expressed in gastric surface epithelial cells, mediates Cl^-/HCO_3^- exchange and is inhibited by NH_4^+. *American Journal of Physiology. Cell Physiology*, **289** (2), C493–C505.

72 Aoyama, F. and Sawaguchi, A. (2011) Functional transformation of gastric parietal cells and intracellular trafficking of ion channels/transporters in the apical canalicular membrane associated with acid secretion. *Biological & Pharmaceutical Bulletin*, **34**, 813–816.

73 Oh, D.S., Wang, H.S., Ohning, G.V. and Pisegna, J.R. (2006) Validation of a new endoscopic technique to assess acid output in Zollinger-Ellison Syndrome. *Clinical Gastroenterology and Hepatology*, **4**, 1467–1473.

74 Dalenbäck, J., Fändriks, L., Olbe, L. and Sjövall, H. (1996) Mechanisms behind changes in gastric acid and bicarbonate outputs during the human interdigestive motility cycle. *American Journal of Physiology – Gastrointestinal and Liver Physiology*, **270**, G113–G122.

75 Zhu, H., Hart, C.A., Sales, D. and Roberts, N.B. (2006) Bacterial killing in gastric juice - effect of pH and pepsin on *Escherichia coli* and *Helicobacter pylori*. *Journal of Medical Microbiology*, **55**, 1265–1270.

76 Etherington, D.J. and Taylor, W.H. (1967) Nomenclature of the pepsins. *Nature*, **216**, 279–280.

77 Agreus, L., Kuipers, E.J., Kupcinskas, L. *et al.* (2012) Rationale in diagnosis and screening of atrophic gastritis with stomach-specific plasma markers. *Scandinavian Journal of Gastroenterology*, **47**, 136–1347.

78 Di Mario, F., Ingegnoli, A., Altavilla, N. *et al.* (2005) Influence of antisecretory treatment with proton pump inhibitors on serum pepsinogen I levels. *Fundamental and Clinical Pharmacology*, **19**, 497–501.

79 Gatta, L., Di Mario, F., Vaira, D. *et al.* (2011) Quantification of serum levels of pepsinogens and gastrin to assess eradication of *Helicobacter pylori*. *Clinical Gastroenterology and Hepatology*, **9**, 440–442.

80 Palileo, C. and Kaunitz, J.D. (2011) Gastrointestinal defense mechanisms. *Current Opinion in Gastroenterology*, **27**, 543–548.

81 Laine, L., Takeuchi, K. and Tarnawski, A. (2008) Gastric mucosal defense and cytoprotection: bench to bedside. *Gastroenterology*, **135**, 41–60.

82 Schubert, M.L. and Kaunitz, J. (2010) Gastric secretion, in *Sleisenger & Fordtran's Gastrointestinal and Liver Disease*, 9th edn (eds M. Feldman, L.S. Friedman and L.J. Brandt), pp. 817–832.

83 Takeuchi, K., Koyama, M., Hayashi, S. and Aihara, E. (2010) Prostaglandin EP receptor subtypes involved in regulating HCO_3^- secretion from gastroduodenal mucosa. *Current Pharmaceutical Design*, **16**, 1241–1251.

84 Ae, T., Ohno, T., Hattori, Y. *et al.* (2010) Role of microsomal prostaglandin E synthase-1 in the facilitation of angiogenesis and the healing of gastric ulcers. *American Journal of Physiology – Gastrointestinal and Liver Physiology*, **299**, G1139–G1146.

85 Schreiber, S. and Scheid, P. (1997) Gastric mucus of the guinea pig: proton carrier and diffusion barrier. *American Journal of Physiology – Gastrointestinal and Liver Physiology*, **272**, G63–G70.

86 Kjellev, S., Nexo, E. and Thim, L. (2006) Systemically administered trefoil factors are secreted into the gastric lumen and increase the viscosity of gastric contents. *British Journal of Pharmacology*, **149**, 92–99.

87 Florkiewicz, R.Z., Ahluwalia, A., Sandor, Z. and Tarnawski, A.S. (2011) Gastric mucosal injury activates bFGF gene expression and triggers preferential translation of high molecular weight bFGF isoforms through CUG-initiated, non-canonical codons. *Biochemical and Biophysical Research Communications*, **409**, 494–499.

88 Marchbank, T., Mahmood, A., Harten, S. *et al.* (2011) Dimethyloxalyglycine stimulates the early stages of gastrointestinal repair processes through VEGF-dependent mechanisms. *Laboratory Investigation*, **91**, 1684–1694.

89 Uc, A., Zhu, X. and Wagner, B.A. (2012) Heme-oxygenase-1 is protective against nonsteroidal anti-inflammatory drug-induced gastric ulcers. *Journal of Pediatric Gastroenterology and Nutrition*, **54**, 471–476.

90 Rossmann, H., Sonnentag, T., Heinzmann, A. *et al.* (2001) Differential expression and regulation of Na^+/H^+ exchanger isoforms in rabbit parietal and mucus cells. *American Journal of Physiology – Gastrointestinal and Liver Physiology*, **281**, G447–G458.

91 Luo, XJ., Li, N.S., Zhang, Y.S. *et al.* (2011) Vanillyl nonanoate protects rat gastric mucosa from ethanol-induced injury through a mechanism involving calcitonin gene-related peptide. *European Journal of Pharmacology*, **666**, 211–217.

92 Chavez-Pina, A.E., Tapia-Alvarez, G.R., Reyes-Raminrez, A. and Navarrete, A. (2011) Carbenoxolone gastroprotective mechanism: participation of nitric oxide/(c) GMP/K(ATP) pathway in ethanol-induced gastric injury in rat. *Fundamental & Clinical Pharmacology*, **25**, 717–722.

93 Fiorucci, S., Distrutti, E., Cirino, G. and Wallace, J.L. (2006) The emerging roles of hydrogen sulfide in the gastrointestinal tract and liver. *Gastroenterology*, **131**, 259–271.

94 Feldman, M. and Richardson, C.T. (1986) Role of thought, sight, smell and taste of food in the cephalic phase of gastric acid secretion in humans. *Gastroenterology*, **90**, 428–433.

95 Vuyyuru, L., Harrington, L., Arimura, A. and Schubert, M.L. (1997) Reciprocal inhibitory paracrine pathways link histamine and somatostatin secretion in the fundus of the stomach. *American Journal of Physiology – Gastrointestinal and Liver Physiology*, **273**, G106–G111.

96 Vuyyuru, L. and Schubert, M.L. (1997) Histamine, acting via H_3 receptors, inhibits somatostatin and stimulates acid secretion in isolated mouse stomach. *Gastroenterology*, **113**, 1545–1552.

97 Sandvik, A.K. and Waldum, H.L. (1991) CCK-B (gastrin) receptor regulates gastric hista-mine release and acid secretion. *American Journal of Physiology – Gastrointestinal and Liver Physiology*, **260**, G925–G928.

98 Schubert, M.L., Saffouri, B., Walsh, J.H. and Makhlouf, G.M. (1985) Inhibition of neurally mediated gastrin secretion by bombesin antiserum. *American Journal of Physiology – Gastrointestinal and Liver Physiology*, **248**, G546–G562.

Answers

1 D
2 C
3 B (oxyntic atrophy)
4 C

CHAPTER 6

Structure and function
of the exocrine pancreas

James H. Grendell

School of Medicine, State University of New York at Stony Brook, Stony Brook, NY, USA
Division of Gastroenterology, Hepatology & Nutrition, Winthrop University Hospital, Mineola, NY, USA

Overview

The exocrine pancreas is the master digestive gland of the body, secreting more than
1 l of clear, bicarbonate-rich fluid into the small intestine each day. This fluid, often
called pancreatic juice, contains digestive enzymes necessary for the hydrolysis of
dietary macronutrients (protein, starch, fat) and fat-soluble vitamin esters into
smaller molecules. Some of these molecules are modified by bile constituents or
intestinal brush border enzymes before all of them are absorbed by enterocytes.

Activation of pancreatic digestive enzymes within the pancreas potentially
may cause "autodigestion" of the gland and acute pancreatitis. For this reason,
the pancreas has mechanisms to prevent premature enzyme activation and, if it
occurs, to contain it.

Gross anatomy

The pancreas is a soft, elongated organ that, in the adult, is 12–20 cm long and
weighs 70–120 g. The pancreatic head lies to the right of the midline, apposed to
the curvature of the duodenum. Its body and tail extend obliquely cephalad posterior to the stomach toward the hilum of the spleen. The common bile duct
enters the head of the pancreas posteriorly and passes through the pancreatic
parenchyma before joining the main pancreatic duct to empty into the small
intestine through the duodenal (major) papilla (Figure 6.1) [1–3].

The main pancreatic duct (duct of Wirsung) arises in the tail of the pancreas and becomes progressively larger as it is joined by branch ducts along its
course through the body and head of the gland to the ampulla of Vater and
major papilla. The accessory duct of Santorini empties through the minor
papilla, which is located in the second portion of the duodenum proximal to

Gastrointestinal Anatomy and Physiology: The Essentials, First Edition. Edited by John F. Reinus and Douglas Simon.
© 2014 John Wiley & Sons, Ltd. Published 2014 by John Wiley & Sons, Ltd.
www.wiley.com/go/reinus/gastro/anatomy

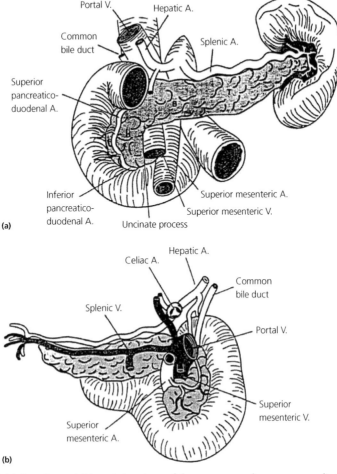

Figure 6.1 (a) Anterior and (b) posterior views of the pancreas and some surrounding structures. A, artery; B, body; H, head; T, tail; V, vein. From Reference [3]. Reproduced with permission of Elsevier.

the duodenal papilla. The accessory duct usually is patent and communicates with the main pancreatic duct (Figure 6.2). In approximately 10% of individuals, the duct of Santorini (arising from the embryonic dorsal pancreas) and the duct of Wirsung (arising from the embryonic ventral pancreas) fail to fuse during embryologic development, an anatomic variation known as pancreas divisum. In such cases, secretions from the body and tail of the pancreas empty through the smaller minor papilla, whereas only secretions from the head and uncinate process of the pancreas empty through the ampulla of Vater and major papilla [5, 6].

The pancreas has a rich arterial blood supply derived from interconnected branches of the celiac and the superior mesenteric arteries (supplying the head

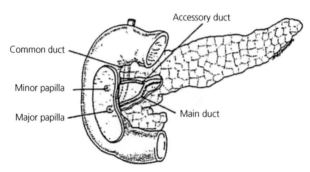

Figure 6.2 Diagrammatic view of the pancreas showing the main and accessory ducts, common bile duct, and major and minor duodenal papillae. From Reference [4]. Reproduced with permission of Elsevier.

and part of the body of the gland) and the splenic artery (supplying the rest of the body and the tail). Venous drainage from the pancreas enters the portal venous system, joining either the portal or splenic veins.

The pancreatic lymphatics generally follow the course of the arteries and veins, with most lymphatic drainage entering the pancreaticosplenic lymph nodes that, in turn, drain into the celiac nodes. Some of the lymphatic drainage enters the pancreaticoduodenal and preaortic nodes. The pancreatic lymphatics interconnect extensively with those from nearby organs and the retroperitoneum.

The sympathetic and parasympathetic efferent innervation of the pancreas is supplied by the vagus and splanchnic nerves by way of the hepatic and celiac plexi. The vagal parasympathetic efferent fibers pass through these plexi but do not synapse until they reach the parasympathetic ganglia in the pancreatic interlobular septa. The postganglionic fibers then innervate the acini, ducts, and islets of Langerhans. Sympathetic nerves arise from the lateral gray matter of the thoracic spinal cord and pass through the greater splanchnic nerves to synapse in the celiac ganglia. Postganglionic fibers follow the distribution of the hepatic, splenic, and superior mesenteric arteries to innervate pancreatic blood vessels. Visceral afferent fibers (which mediate pain) travel through the vagus nerve to the celiac ganglia and splanchnic nerves to reach the thoracic sympathetic chain and the spinal root ganglia.

Microscopic anatomy

The pancreas is formed of lobules surrounded by connective tissue septae containing blood vessels, lymphatics, nerves, and exocrine secretory ducts. The lobular parenchyma consists mainly of acini involved in exocrine secretion (>80% of the gland) (Figure 6.3). Scattered among the acini are the islets of Langerhans (1–2% of the gland), which are responsible for pancreatic endocrine secretion [7].

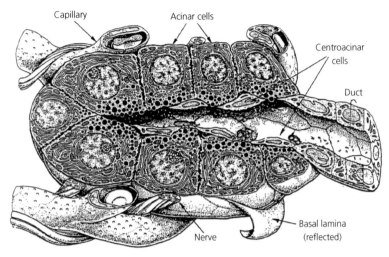

Figure 6.3 Histologic organization of the pancreatic acinus and its relationship to surrounding capillaries and nerves. From Reference [7]. Reproduced with permission of Elsevier.

Acinar cells are tall and pyramidal and are situated on a basal lamina. They are highly specialized for the synthesis, storage, and secretion of large amounts of protein, mainly in the form of digestive enzymes. In the resting state, the apical portion of the acinar cell is filled with eosinophilic zymogen granules about 1 µm in diameter. After ingestion of a meal or administration of a secretagogue, protein secretion by acinar cells is accompanied by a rapid decrease in both the size and number of zymogen granules. The basal portion of the acinar cell contains the nucleus and extensive rough ER and is separated from the zymogen granules by a highly developed Golgi complex. The apices of the acinar cells converge on a central lumen continuous with a duct lined with flattened centroacinar cells that contain relatively few organelles and no secretory granules. Around each acinus lies a rich capillary network and nerve fibers that terminate adjacent to the acinar cells.

The acini empty into intralobular ducts lined by cuboidal epithelium. These then join to form interlobular ducts that empty into the main pancreatic duct. The larger ducts, lined primarily by tall columnar cells with occasional goblet and argentaffin cells, are accompanied by arterial and venous blood vessels and nerves and are surrounded by connective tissue.

Casts formed by retrograde injection of the pancreatic duct system with silicon demonstrate that the organization of ducts and acini is complex. Acini are *not* merely spherical units at the ends of the duct system, similar to a bunch of grapes on a stem. Rather, acini are commonly curved, branching tubules that anastomose, occasionally loop, and ultimately end blindly [8].

Stellate cells similar to hepatic stellate cells have been identified in the pancreas. In the quiescent state, these cells contain fat storage globules. When activated, however, they undergo a marked morphologic change to resemble myofibroblasts and express genes for collagen synthesis. In the liver, stellate cells are the major cell type responsible for synthesis of extracellular collagen and are believed to play a critical role in the development of fibrosis in response to liver injury. It is likely that stellate cells function similarly in the pancreas and are responsible for the fibrosis observed in chronic pancreatitis and the desmoplastic reaction seen in pancreatic cancer [9].

The endocrine pancreas consists of about one million round or oval islets of Langerhans, each about 0.2 mm in diameter. They are separated from the surrounding exocrine tissue by fine fibers of connective tissue. The most common types of islet cells are the insulin-secreting beta cell (in the center of the islet) and the glucagon-secreting alpha cell (in the periphery). The other major cell types are the SST-secreting delta cell and the PP-secreting PP cell.

Each islet is surrounded by a glomerulus-like network of capillaries lined by fenestrated endothelium. After perfusing the islet, efferent blood from this capillary network bathes surrounding exocrine tissue. The islet cell blood vessels, therefore, form an insuloacinar portal system. Other arterioles carry blood directly to acinar tissue without passing through islets. The result of the insulo-acinar portal system is that acini surrounding islets (peri-insular acini) are exposed to much higher levels of islet hormones (e.g., insulin, glucagon) than more distantly located islets. This likely explains the observation that peri-insular acini have larger cells and nuclei and more zymogen granules (with different enzyme composition) than other acini [10].

Pancreatic juice

Water and electrolytes

Pancreatic juice is a clear, alkaline fluid that is isosmotic with plasma. Water moves into pancreatic juice passively along osmotic gradients [11]. The major cations in pancreatic juice are Na^+ and K^+, which are secreted at concentrations similar to their plasma concentrations and independent of the rate of juice secretion. Although the total anion concentration of pancreatic juice does not vary with its secretory rate, the amounts of the major anions, HCO_3^- and Cl^-, do. At low rates of juice secretion, the concentration of HCO_3^- is about 30–60 mmol/l but rises to about 140 mmol/l at high secretory rates, with a corresponding reciprocal decrease in Cl^- concentration (Figure 6.4).

This flow-related reciprocal relationship of HCO_3^- and Cl^- concentrations in pancreatic juice is due to the relative contributions of acinar and ductal epithelial cell secretions. At low rates of juice secretion in the fasting or interdigestive state (about 0.2 ml/min), much of the pancreatic juice comes from acinar cells with anion concentrations similar to those of plasma. Following stimulation of the pancreas by a meal, however, the secretory rate rises to about 4.0 ml/min and predominately consists of bicarbonate-rich fluid secreted by ductal epithelial cells.

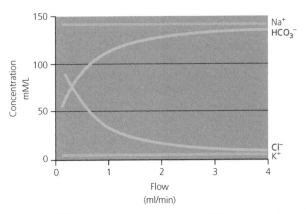

Figure 6.4 Concentrations of the major ions in pancreatic juice. The concentrations of Na^+ and K^+ are similar to those in plasma and do not change with increasing rates of secretion. However, as the rate of secretion rises, the concentration of HCO_3^- increases substantially coupled with a reciprocal decrease in the concentration of Cl^-. From Reference [12]. Reproduced with permission of Morgan & Claypool Life Sciences.

Pancreatic bicarbonate is essential to the digestive process, neutralizing gastric acid in the duodenum and raising the duodenal and jejunal pH so that pancreatic digestive enzymes and bile salts are active. Pancreatic digestive enzymes function optimally at a neutral to slightly alkaline pH and are progressively inactivated and ultimately irreversibly denatured as the pH becomes more acidic. Bile salts precipitate at low pH.

In addition to the four major cations and anions mentioned earlier, pancreatic juice contains other electrolytes: Ca^{2+} (1–2 mEq/l) and minute amounts of Mg^{2+}, Zn^{2+}, HPO_4^{-2}, and SO_4^{-2}.

Proteins

Human pancreatic juice has a protein concentration of approximately 1–10%. Most of these proteins are cofactors and digestive enzymes, including 20 isoforms of 12 different enzymes. Pancreatic juice also contains pancreatic secretory trypsin inhibitor and very small amounts of plasma proteins and glycoproteins [13].

The three major categories of digestive enzymes in pancreatic juice are proteases, which digest proteins and peptides and comprise about 75% of juice proteins by weight; amylase, which digests starch; and lipases, which digest triglycerides and phospholipids (Table 6.1). In addition, pancreatic juice contains colipase, a peptide cofactor that contributes to lipolysis by binding to bile salt–lipid surfaces, enhancing the ability of lipase to digest triglycerides. All of the proteases and also phospholipase and colipase are secreted by the pancreas as inactive proenzymes (zymogens). After reaching the duodenal lumen, trypsinogen is converted to trypsin by the brush border enzyme enterokinase, which cleaves the trypsinogen activation peptide, exposing trypsin's catalytic

Table 6.1 Sites of action of pancreatic digestive enzymes.

Enzyme	Substrate	Sites of action	Products
Amylase	Carbohydrates (amylase, amylopectin, glycogen)	α-1,4 linkage between hexoses (but not at branch points or endpoints)	Maltose, maltotriose, α-limit dextrins
Endopeptidases (trypsin, chymotrypsin, elastase)	Proteins, peptides	Internal peptide bonds	Smaller peptides
Exopeptidases (carboxypeptidases)	Proteins, peptides	Peptide bonds at carboxyl terminal	Terminal amino acid plus remainder of protein or peptide
Lipase	Triglycerides	Ester linkage of fatty acid in position 1	Fatty acid, monoglycerides
Phospholipase	Phospholipids (lecithin)	Ester linkage in position 2	Fatty acid, 1,1-diglyceride (e.g., lysolecithin)

domain. Trypsin can then activate the other proenzymes as well as trypsinogen molecules. Amylase, lipase, and ribonucleases are secreted in their active forms.

The acinar cell synthesizes and secretes a trypsin inhibitor, pancreatic secretory trypsin inhibitor, in low concentration. This protein protects the pancreas from damage by premature activation of trypsinogen to trypsin. Once pancreatic juice enters the intestine, however, trypsinogen is activated to trypsin so rapidly and completely that the relatively small amount of trypsin inhibitor in pancreatic juice does not interfere with the normal digestive process.

Cellular mechanisms of secretion

Water and electrolytes
Based on the distribution of aquaporin water channels in the human pancreas, the small intralobular ducts are likely the main pancreatic site of water and electrolyte secretion. The intestinal peptide hormone, secretin, is the most potent stimulus to water and bicarbonate secretion. Secretin binds to receptors on the basolateral duct cell surface and stimulates intracellular cAMP production, resulting in activation of PKA. ACh released from cholinergic nerves potentiates the effects of secretin by binding to a receptor that causes an increase in intracellular calcium concentration.

Bicarbonate is secreted by pancreatic centroacinar and duct cells against large concentration and electrochemical gradients. Bicarbonate ions secreted into the pancreatic duct are formed by hydration of intravascular CO_2 by CA and direct

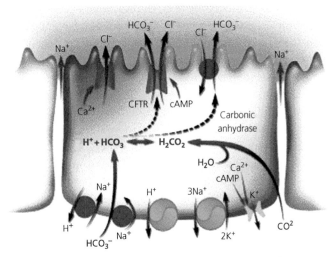

Figure 6.5 Cellular mechanisms involved in the secretion of HCO_3^- by the pancreatic duct cell. HCO_3^- enters the cell via cotransport with Na^+ on the basolateral surface of the cell and is formed by the action of CA on H_2O and CO_2. Secretion is mediated by secretin which increases intracellular cAMP and ACh which increases intracellular Ca^{2+}. Cl^- enters the duct lumen through conductance channels provided by CFTR (mediated by cAMP) and a Ca^+-mediated channel. HCO_3^- is secreted into the duct lumen in exchange for Cl^-. HCO_3^- may also pass into the duct lumen via CFTR and the Ca^+-mediated conductance, at least under some circumstances. Na^+ travels into the duct lumen by electrodiffusion through paracellular tight junction channels, and water enters through aquaporin water channels (not shown). From Reference [12]. Reproduced with permission of Morgan & Claypool Life Sciences.

uptake of HCO_3^- by means of a basolateral Na^+/HCO_3^- cotransporter. Chloride is secreted into the duct lumen by activation of both a cAMP-dependent chloride channel (the CFTR) and a calcium-dependent channel on the apical duct cell surface. The resulting high concentration of Cl^- in the duct lumen allows exchange of Cl^- for HCO_3^- through a Cl^-/HCO_3^- antiport. Recent experimental evidence suggests that CFTR and the calcium-dependent chloride channel may contribute to bicarbonate secretion by also serving as bicarbonate conductance channels, at least under some circumstances. Cations, mainly Na^+, are secreted by electrodiffusion through paracellular tight junction channels. Water is secreted through aquaporin water channels (Figure 6.5) [14].

Proteins

The proteins secreted by the exocrine pancreas, primarily digestive enzymes, are synthesized on ribosomes of the rough ER in acinar cells. Newly synthesized proteins enter the cisternal space of the ER by insertion of a lipophilic "signal" or "leader" sequence of amino acids at the amino-terminal end of each protein into the membrane [15]. These proteins may undergo modifications and conformational changes in the ER before they are transported in transition vesicles to the Golgi complex.

Additional posttranslational processing (e.g., glycosylation, peptide cleavage) occurs there. The Golgi complex also plays a key role in sorting and targeting newly formed proteins so that they reach the appropriate cellular compartment (e.g., digestive enzymes to zymogen granules, lysosomal enzymes to lysosomes). The final mixture of secretory proteins buds from the Golgi complex to form condensing vacuoles that ultimately become zymogen granules, the storage form of digestive enzymes and other secretory proteins [16]. In zymogen granules, secreted proteins are arranged in a tightly packed, crystalline-like state [17]. Zymogen granules move toward the apices of acinar cells by a process involving microtubules.

Stimulation of acinar-cell protein secretion is due to specific binding of ACh and, at least in some species, of the intestinal peptide hormone CCK to GPCRs on the basolateral cell surface. Receptor binding begins an intracellular cascade of events. First, PLC is activated by a G-protein-mediated mechanism. Then, PLC cleaves phosphatidylinositol to inositol 1,4,5-trisphosphate (IP$_3$) and 1,2-diacylglycerol (DAG). IP$_3$ causes release of calcium from intracytoplasmic stores and a rapid but transient spike in cytosolic calcium concentration that appears as a "wave" that propagates from the apical to the basolateral cell surface. Each of these calcium oscillations results in zymogen granule exocytosis and pancreatic enzyme secretion into the lumen. Protein kinase C is activated by DAG, and calcium binds to calmodulin to activate several additional protein kinases and a protein phosphatase. These protein kinases and phosphatases likely play a role in initiating and regulating exocytosis [18].

Exocytosis involves fusion of the zymogen granule membrane with the apical cell membrane, enabling release of granule contents into the acinar lumen. Because of the limited apical surface area, the rate of exocytosis observed following stimulation of acinar cells suggests that zymogen granules also fuse with each other to allow exocytosis of zymogen granules deep in the cell through granules closer to or at the apical cell membrane. This complex process is mediated by specialized proteins called *SNARE* proteins, calmodulin-dependent protein kinases, and interactions of actin and myosin [19].

Acinar cells also have secretin receptors on their basolateral surface. Just as in duct cells, binding of secretin to its acinar-cell receptor results in an increase of cAMP and activation of PKA. Secretin can potentiate the effects of ACh and CCK on pancreatic enzyme secretion, at least in some species.

Regulation of pancreatic secretion

Basal secretion

During the human interdigestive or fasting state, the volume of pancreatic juice secreted into the duodenum is low. Enzyme secretion is approximately 10% of maximal and bicarbonate secretion only 2% of maximal. Brief periods of increased pancreatic enzyme and bicarbonate secretion occur every 60–120 min in association with the increased intestinal motor activity of phase III of the interdigestive MMCs [20]. Cholinergic neural input is the primary regulator of increased motor and secretory activity during phase III; motilin secretion from duodenal endocrine cells appears to play a role in its initiation. Alpha-adrenergic tone acts as an inhibitor of pancreatic secretion in the fasting state.

Postprandial secretion

After ingestion of a meal, the exocrine pancreas secretes enzymes and bicarbonate at approximately 60–75% of the levels attained after intravenous infusions of maximally effective doses of secretagogues such as secretin and CCK [21]. This meal-related regulation of secretion can be understood as having cephalic, gastric, and intestinal phases, although considerable overlap between phases exists.

The cephalic phase is stimulated by the thought, sight, taste, or smell of food. It is primarily regulated by vagal cholinergic innervation and accounts for about 25% of meal-stimulated secretion. The gastric phase is produced by distension of the stomach, which activates vago-vagal reflexes. It accounts for only about 10% of meal-stimulated pancreatic secretion. By determining the rate of entry of acid and nutrients into the duodenum, however, gastric emptying strongly influences the intestinal phase, the predominant phase in the pancreatic response to a meal.

During the intestinal phase of pancreatic secretion, duodenal acidification causes release of secretin, which binds to receptors on pancreatic ductal epithelial cells. Intraduodenal fatty acids and bile may also stimulate secretin release. The rise in plasma secretin concentration after a meal (potentiated by vagal cholinergic stimulation) is responsible for a marked increase in pancreatic water and bicarbonate output.

Digestive enzyme secretion is stimulated by the presence of fatty acids, oligopeptides, amino acids, and calcium in the intestine. They cause duodenal CCK release into the circulation and activation of cholinergic enteropancreatic reflexes that stimulate pancreatic enzyme secretion. Inasmuch as studies of human pancreatic tissue have failed to identify CCK-A receptors (high-affinity, secretion-stimulating receptors) on acinar cells, it is likely that CCK stimulates pancreatic secretion in humans by binding to afferent sensory vagal neurons and intrapancreatic cholinergic neurons rather than directly to acinar cells.

The human pancreas has the ability to synthesize and secrete substantially more digestive enzymes than are required to meet normal demands. An increase in fecal fat excretion (steatorrhea) does not occur until the pancreas has lost at least 90% of its exocrine secretory capacity [22].

CCK and secretin-releasing factors
and feedback regulation

The meal-stimulated secretion of CCK and secretin by duodenal mucosal endocrine cells is caused, at least in part, by releasing factors produced in the duodenum and secreted into the lumen in response to the presence of peptides (for CCK-releasing factors) and acid (for secretin-releasing factors) [23, 24]. Releasing factors for CCK and secretin may also be contained in pancreatic juice. These factors are susceptible to proteolytic inactivation by the pancreatic enzymes, trypsin, chymotrypsin, and elastase. When there is no food in the duodenum to act as a substrate for pancreatic proteases, these enzymes destroy the releasing factors for CCK and secretin, resulting in feedback inhibition of secretion.

Feedback inhibition of pancreatic secretion by intraduodenal proteases such as trypsin, chymotrypsin, and elastase has been demonstrated in the rat; several studies suggest that bile salts also sometimes may inhibit secretion. More limited data in humans support the existence of feedback inhibition of pancreatic digestive enzyme secretion by intraduodenal proteases through a process mediated by cholinergic nerves. The importance of mechanism in either normal physiology or disease remains to be determined.

Another form of feedback inhibition of pancreatic exocrine secretion results from neutralization of gastric acid in the duodenum by pancreatic bicarbonate. This causes an increase in duodenal pH, removing the primary stimulus for release of secretin by the small intestine and producing a negative feedback effect on pancreatic water and bicarbonate secretion.

Inhibitors of pancreatic secretion

Postprandial exocrine secretion by the pancreas reaches only 60–75% of the maximal levels attained when pharmacologic concentrations of secretagogues are administered to human subjects [21, 23]. This suggests the existence of physiologic inhibitory mechanisms. The pancreatic islet cell peptides glucagon, PP, and SST (also released from the intestine) have all been suggested as possible mediators of such inhibitory processes.

Another potential candidate is PYY, found in ileal and colonic endocrine cells and released in response to the intraluminal presence of lipid. PYY, and possibly other factors such as GLP-1, may act as an "ileal brake" to reduce pancreatic secretion after digestion of a meal has been largely completed. It is likely that most inhibitors of pancreatic exocrine secretion act primarily by altering cholinergic transmission. SST, the most potent inhibitor, however, appears to act in multiple sites.

Effects of pancreatic blood flow

Although ingestion of a meal increases overall splanchnic blood flow, postprandial changes in pancreatic blood flow have not been extensively studied, particularly in unanesthetized subjects. Physiologic levels of stimulation (due to administration of CCK or secretin or due to duodenal acidification) in several canine studies [24–26] did not appear to increase total pancreatic perfusion. This indicates that, under physiologic conditions, pancreatic secretion may not be limited by blood flow.

Table 6.2 Protective mechanisms to prevent pancreatic autodigestion.

- The potentially most dangerous pancreatic digestive enzymes are secreted as inactive proenzymes (zymogens)
- Prior to secretion, digestive enzymes are separated from the rest of the acinar cell in membrane-bound secretory granules (zymogen granules)
- The enzyme enterokinase which initiates the activation of the pancreatic digestive proenzymes is located on the intestinal brush border, physically separate from the pancreas
- A pancreatic secretory trypsin inhibitor is present in the zymogen granule, which can inactivate small amounts of trypsin if premature activation occurs within the acinar cell
- The pancreatic duct cells secrete large amounts of fluid to flush digestive enzymes out of the pancreas and into the duodenum

Protective mechanisms

The premature activation of trypsinogen to trypsin within acinar cells or pancreatic ducts can lead to activation of pancreatic proenzymes, initiating an autodigestive process (acute pancreatitis) that can have devastating effects on the pancreas and other organs. A number of mechanisms have evolved to protect the pancreas from this eventuality (Table 6.2).

Multiple choice questions

The enzyme responsible for the activation of pancreatic zymogens (inactive proenzymes) in the small intestine is:
- A Cholecystokinin
- B Trypsinogen activation peptide
- C Pancreatic polypeptide
- D Enterokinase
- E Elastase

1 Which of the following plays a major role in the exocytosis of pancreatic digestive enzymes from acinar cells?
- A Intracellular calcium oscillations
- B Increased intracellular cyclic AMP
- C Activation of the cystic fibrosis transmembrane conductance regulator
- D Trypsinogen activation to trypsin in zymogen granules
- E Bicarbonate/chloride exchange across the zymogen granule membrane

2 In humans, stimulation of pancreatic enzyme secretion by cholecystokinin:
- A Requires insulin from the insuloacinar portal system
- B Mediates the cephalic phase of secretion
- C Can be inhibited by administration of atropine
- D Effects only proteases
- E Results in the appearance of more zymogen granules in acinar cells

3 A clinical test of pancreatic exocrine function involves injecting secretin intravenously into a subject while measuring the concentration of a substance in fluid aspirated from the subject's duodenum both before and after secretin injection. Measurement of which of the following would be most useful in assessing pancreatic function using this test?
- A Sodium
- B Potassium

C Calcium

D Chloride

E Bicarbonate

4 Which of the following is most important in helping to protect the pancreatic acinar cell against autodigestion?

A Carbonic anhydrase

B Pancreatic secretory trypsin inhibitor

C Calcium oscillations

D The "ileal brake" function of peptide YY

E Stellate cell activation

5 Concerning pancreatic physiology, which statement is *false*?

A As the rate of pancreatic secretion increases, the concentration of chloride decreases and bicarbonate increases.

B Pancreatic enzymes function best at a neutral pH.

C Pancreatic acinar cells produce digestive enzymes and the duct cells produce fluid and electrolytes.

D CCK stimulates the acinar cells and secretin stimulates the ductal cells.

E All the digestive pancreatic enzymes are released in an inactive form and activated in the duodenum.

6 The duodenal mucosal enzyme responsible for activating pancreatic proteases is:

A Pepsinogen

B Enterokinase

C Trypsinogen

D Phospholipase A2

E CCK (cholecystokinin)

References

1 Basmajian, J.V. (1980) *Grant's Method of Anatomy*, 10th edn, Williams and Wilkins, Baltimore, pp. 170–173.

2 Clemente, C.D. (1985) *Gray's Anatomy of the Human Body*, 30th edn, Lea& Febiger, Philadelphia, pp. 1502–1507.

3 Grendell, J.H. (1995) Embryology, anatomy, and anomalies of the pancreas, in *Bockus Gastroenterology*, 5th edn (eds W.S. Haubrich, F. Schaffner, and J.E. Berk), WB Saunders, Philadelphia, p. 2816.

4 Grendell, J.H. (1995) Embryology, anatomy, and anomalies of the pancreas, in *Bockus Gastroenterology*, 5th edn (eds W.S. Haubrich, F. Schaffner and J.E. Berk), WB Saunder, Philadelphia, p. 2815.

5 Kleitsch, W.P. (1955) Anatomy of the pancreas. A study with special reference to the duct system. *Archives of Surgery*, **71**, 795–802.

6 Kreel, L. (1975) Pancreatic duct caliber and variations on autopsy pancreatography, in *Efficiency and Limits of Radiologic Examinations of the Pancreas* (ed. H. Anacker),Publishing Sciences Group, Acton, pp. 214–217.

7 Fawcett, D.W. (1986) *Bloom and Fawcett: A Textbook of Histology*, 11th edn,WB Saunders Company, Philadelphia, pp. 716–730.

8 Bockman, D.E., Boydston, W.R. and Parsa, I. (1983) Architecture of human pancreas: implications for early changes in pancreatic disease. *Gastroenterology*, **85**, 55–61.

9 Erkan, M., Adler, G., Apte, M.V. *et al.* (2012) StellaTUM: current consensus and discussion on pancreatic stellate cell research. *Gut*, **61**, 172–178.

10 Williams, J.A. and Goldfine, I.D. (1985) The insulin-pancreatic acinar axis. *Diabetes*, **34**, 980–986.

11 Domschke, S., Domschke, W., Rosch, W. *et al.* (1976) Bicarbonate and cyclic AMP content of pure human pancreatic juice in response to graded doses of synthetic secretin. *Gastroenterology*, **70**, 533–536.

12 Pandol, S.J. (2010) *The Exocrine Pancreas*, Morgan & Claypool Life Sciences, San Rafael.

13 Scheele, G., Bartelt, D. and Bieger, W. (1981) Characterization of human exocrine pancreatic proteins by two-dimensional isoelectric focusing/sodium dodecyl sulfate gel electrophoresis. *Gastroenterology*, **80**, 461–473.

14 Steward, M.C., Ishiguro, H. and Case, R.M. (2005) Mechanisms of bicarbonate secretion in the pancreatic duct. *Annual Review of Physiology*, **67**, 377–409.

15 Blobel, G. (2000) Protein targeting. *Chembiochem*, **1**, 86–103.

16 Case, R.M. (1978) Synthesis, intracellular transport and discharge of exportable proteins in the pancreatic acinar cell and other cells. *Biological Reviews of the Cambridge Philosophical Society*, **53**, 211–354.

17 Rothman, S.S., Iskander, N., Attwood, D. *et al.* (1989) The interior of a whole and unmodified biological object—the zymogen granule—viewed with a high resolution x-ray microscope. *Biochimica et Biophysica Acta*, **991**, 484–486.

18 Williams, J.A. (2001) Intracellular signaling mechanisms activated by cholecystokinin-regulating synthesis and secretion of digestive enzymes. *Annual Review of Physiology*, **63**, 77–97.

19 Pickett, J.A., Campos-Toimil, M., Thomas, P., and Edwardson, J.M. (2007) Identification of SNAREs that mediate zymogen granule exocytosis. *Biochemical and Biophysical Research Communications*, **359**, 599–603.

20 Keller, J. and Layer, P. (2002) Circadian pancreatic enzyme pattern and relationship between secretory and motor activities in fasting humans. *Journal of Applied Physiology*, **93**, 592–600.

21 Keller, J. and Layer, P. (2005) Human pancreatic exocrine response to nutrients in health and disease. *Gut*, **54**, 1–28.

22 DiMagno, E.P., Go, V.L.W. and Summerskill, W.H.J. (2008) Relations between pancreatic enzyme outputs and malabsorption in severe pancreatic insufficiency. *The New England Journal of Medicine*, **288**, 813–815.

23 Morriset, J. (2008) Negative control of human pancreatic secretion: physiological mechanisms and factors. *Pancreas*, **37**, 1–12.

24 Wang, Y., Prpic, V., Green, G.M. *et al.* Luminal CCK-releasing factor stimulates CCK release from human intestinal endocrine and STC-1 cells. *American Journal of Physiology - Gastrointestinal and Liver Physiology*, **282**, G16–G22.

25 Aune, S. and Semb, L.S. (1969) The effect of secretin and pancreozymin on pancreatic blood flow in the conscious and anesthetized dog. *Acta Physiologica Scandinavica*, **76**, 406–414.

26 Beijer, H.J.M., Brouwer, F.A.S. and Charbon, G.A. Time course and sensitivity of secretin-stimulated pancreatic secretion and blood flow in the anesthetized dog. *Scandinavian Journal of Gastroenterology*, **14**, 295–300.

Answers

1 D
2 A
3 C
4 E
5 B
6 E
7 B

CHAPTER 7

Absorption and secretion of fluid and electrolytes

Lawrence R. Schiller

Dallas Campus, Texas A&M College of Medicine, Dallas, TX, USA
Digestive Health Associates of Texas, Dallas, TX, USA
Baylor University Medical Center, Dallas, TX, USA

Introduction

Approximately 10 l of ingested liquid and secretions enter the intestine each day, but only 100 ml of water are excreted in stool, an absorptive efficiency of 99% [1]. The maximum intestinal water-absorptive capacity is theoretically even greater, perhaps as much as 30 l per day, a rate that exceeds the excretory ability of the kidneys. In illness, absorptive capacity can decrease; even a reduction of absorptive efficiency of 1–2% can result in diarrhea, and more substantial reductions can produce life-threatening dehydration and electrolyte depletion. An understanding of the normal physiology and pathophysiology of intestinal water and electrolyte absorption is essential to the management of diarrheal diseases.

All organisms must extract needed raw materials from the environment. Unicellular organisms and simple multicellular organisms have sufficient external surface areas to do this without dedicated specialized structures. The external surface areas of more complex creatures, however, are insufficient to absorb materials needed to sustain life. Terrestrial animals face the additional problem that their skins have evolved to protect the internal environment from drying, not as an absorptive surface. Thus, most animals have an internal alimentary tract to handle the essential job of digesting nutrients and absorbing fluid, electrolytes, and nutrients from the environment. The structure of the alimentary tract and its lining cells, the enterocytes, is highly evolved to perform these functions.

Structural considerations

Transport processes necessary to sustain human life require a large surface area. The small intestine, the site of most gut fluid and electrolyte absorption, is a tube roughly 3–6 m long (depending on its contractile state). It is extensively folded

Gastrointestinal Anatomy and Physiology: The Essentials, First Edition. Edited by John F. Reinus and Douglas Simon.
© 2014 John Wiley & Sons, Ltd. Published 2014 by John Wiley & Sons, Ltd.
www.wiley.com/go/reinus/gastro/anatomy

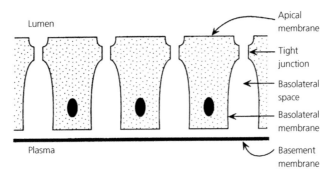

Figure 7.1 Basic arrangement of the gastrointestinal epithelium. Epithelial cells are polarized with distinct apical and basolateral cell membrane domains separated by tight junctions.

and covered by villi making its surface area 15–30-times greater than that of an unfolded cylinder of the same length and diameter. The luminal surface area of both the small intestine and colon is additionally increased 20- to 40-fold by the presence of microvilli on enterocytes. Thus, the total absorptive surface area of the intestine is estimated to be over 200 m², roughly the size of a tennis court [2]. This large surface is required to absorb the fluid, electrolytes, and nutrients needed by a 70-kg human, with some excess capacity to deal with the vagaries of intake, disease, and dysfunction that commonly occur during life.

The enterocytes lining the intestine have structural complexity that facilitates the global function of the intestine (Figure 7.1). Each intestinal cell is polarized, with an apical membrane that faces the lumen and a basolateral membrane that faces the extracellular space, which is in communication with the blood stream. These membrane domains are separated by tight junctions that connect each enterocyte to its neighbors. Different transport proteins are located in different portions of the cell membrane, and thus, the transport properties of the apical and basolateral membranes differ [3].

There are several different types of transport proteins. *Channels* are proteins that create fluid-filled pores in the cell membrane that allow water-soluble (hydrophilic) molecules, such as sodium and chloride ions, to cross the lipid-rich (hydrophobic) cell membrane (Figure 7.2) [4]. Channels often are constructed of protein chains that aggregate to span the membrane and contain a water-filled space within. Channels are ion specific (e.g., for sodium, potassium, or chloride) and are "gated," allowing them to open and close rapidly, thereby constraining the number of ions that can enter the cell. Channels allow ions to cross the plasma membrane down an electrochemical gradient (i.e., from higher to lower concentration) and thus are a mechanism for passive movement across the cell membrane. Channels for water movement (aquaporins) are present in many body organs, but do not appear to be essential to water transport in the intestine [5].

Carriers are proteins that facilitate the movement of specific solutes (e.g., glucose, fructose, and amino acids) across the plasma membrane. The solute may be propelled

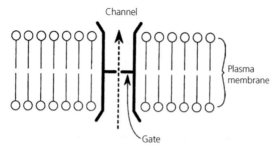

Channel

Plasma membrane

Gate

Figure 7.2 Channels are pores in the cell membrane which are specific for a particular ion with gates that open and close rapidly allowing ions to diffuse down their electrochemical gradients.

by its own concentration gradient (facilitated diffusion) (Figure 7.3a) or by using energy from the concentration gradients of other solutes. When the concentration gradient of another solute is used, the other solute can be moved in the same direction as the solute of interest (cotransport) (Figure 7.3b) or in the opposite direction (exchange) (Figure 7.3c). Although ATP is not consumed directly by the carrier, energy in the form of ATP can produce "secondary active transport" if the concentration gradient for the cotransported or exchanged solute is created by active transport elsewhere in the cell. It is thought that carriers produce their effects by conformational changes that allow cyclic movement across the plasma membrane [1].

Pumps are transport proteins that move ions and other solutes against electrochemical gradients by directly linking energy produced by hydrolysis of ATP to transport (Figure 7.4) [1]. For example, the sodium–potassium ATPase located on the basolateral membranes of enterocytes transports three sodium ions out of the cell in exchange for two potassium ions that enter the cell. This maintains a low sodium concentration and a net negative electrical charge in the interior of the cell but requires energy because the sodium concentration in the fluid outside the cell is so much higher than the intracellular sodium concentration. The sodium gradient produced by this pump can be used to power sodium–nutrient cotransport at the apical enterocyte membrane.

Enterocytes in different regions of the intestine express different transport proteins and thus have different abilities to transport molecules (Table 7.1). The combination of transport abilities in various regions of the intestine is therefore different. There are also important differences in transport capabilities between cells in the crypts and those in the villi. Since the cells in the villi derive from those in the crypts, this implies that differentiation of these cells as they travel from crypt to villus tip includes expression of new transport proteins [6].

The point of division between the apical and the basolateral membranes is the *tight junction*, the place that cells attach to one another. Tight junctions are part of the "apical junction complex" composed of a tight junction, an adherens junction, desmosomes, and gap junctions (from apical to basal) [7]. Tight junctions form regulated and selective permeation pathways for paracellular transport from the

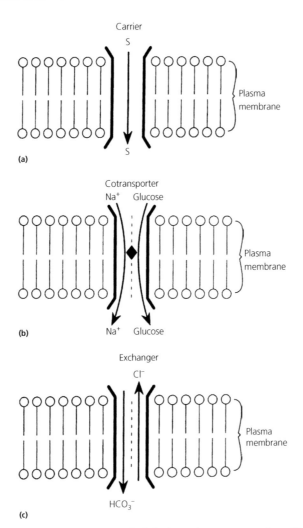

Figure 7.3 Carriers are protein complexes which facilitate the movement of specific solutes across the membrane. The solute may move in response to its own concentration gradient (facilitated diffusion) (panel a) or by using the energy inherent in concentration gradients of other solutes produced by other transporters (secondary active transport). Subtypes include cotransporters (panel b), carriers which move two substances in the same direction across a membrane, and exchangers (panel c), carriers that move ions in opposite directions across a membrane.

lumen to plasma and vice versa. Transmembrane protein particles of claudin form intimate connections between cells in a pattern resembling fingerprints. Intracellular actin filaments attach to the plasma membrane immediately below these strands and also interact with nearby scaffolding proteins, such as ZO-1 and cingulin. Actin and these scaffolding proteins seem to be part of the regulatory apparatus for tight junctions.

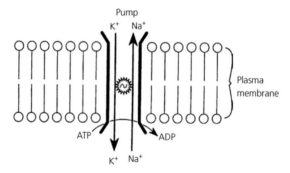

Figure 7.4 Pumps are transport proteins that move solutes against electrochemical gradients by directly linking energy production (i.e., ATP hydrolysis) to transport.

Table 7.1 Some transport proteins of the intestine.

	Jejunum	Ileum	R colon	L colon
Apical transport proteins				
Na channel	+	+	+	+
K channel	?	?	+	+
Cl channel	+	+	?	?
Nutrient–Na cotransporter	+	+	–	–
Glucose, galactose, amino acids				
Na–bile acid cotransporter	–	+	–	–
Na–H exchanger[a]	+	+	+	+
Cl–HCO3 exchanger[a]	–	+	+	+
SCFA–anion exchanger	–	–	+	+
H, K ATPase pump	–	–	–	+
Basolateral transport proteins				
Na, K ATPase pump	+	+	+	+
Na:K:2Cl cotransporter	+	+	+	+
Na–H exchanger	+	+	+	+
K channels	+	+	+	+

[a]Coupling of Na–H and Cl–HCO3 exchangers = electroneutral NaCl entry

Adherens junctions and desmosomes are located deep to tight junctions (farther from the apical cell membrane). They are attached to the cytoskeleton and seem to serve a structural purpose by holding cells together rather than a regulatory one for paracellular transport. Gap junctions are even further from the apical surface and serve as pathways for cell-to-cell signaling by small molecules.

Different amounts and types of tight junction proteins in different parts of the intestine determine the "tightness" and selectivity of the paracellular pathway [7] so that tight junctions in different regions of the intestine vary in their selectivity for different molecules and ions. For example, the tight junctions in the jejunum are characterized as "leaky" (low resistance) pathways and are cation selective, whereas those in the colon are "tighter" and anion selective.

Principles of transepithelial transport

The mucosa forms a barrier between the luminal contents of the intestine and the extracellular space of the body. Transfer of water and solutes between the lumen and the extracellular space is controlled by epithelial properties that vary among the jejunum, ileum, proximal colon, and distal colon [1]. In health, these different regions work together to accomplish the task of absorbing necessary dietary contents in an efficient manner. In disease, the different regions may function abnormally, causing diarrhea, or may minimize diarrhea by compensating for abnormal proximal bowel function.

The basic principle of water movement across the intestinal epithelium is that water moves passively down osmotic or hydraulic pressure gradients [5]. Reduced to basic principles, the intestinal epithelium can be envisioned as functioning as a semipermeable membrane: a membrane that allows solvent molecules to pass freely but prevents the passage of solute. In the case of the intestine, water moves freely to equalize osmotic pressure on either side of the epithelium. Thus, water will leave the lumen when luminal contents are hypotonic to plasma and will enter the lumen when luminal contents are hypertonic.

The intestine is not a perfectly semipermeable membrane, however, because solute can cross from the lumen to plasma or vice versa. Solute transport is accomplished by a variety of mechanisms that vary from region to region of the intestine. These mechanisms include transcellular permeation by means of ion channels, ion exchangers, cotransporters, and molecules in the cell membrane that facilitate diffusion. Paracellular permeation via tight junctions between epithelial cells also is an important mechanism for solute transport, especially in the jejunum [1].

Active transport refers to solute translocation that directly or indirectly requires energy (Figure 7.5) [1]. Hydrolysis of ATP can be used to develop an electrochemical gradient between the lumen, the interior of the cell, and the extracellular space. For instance, sodium–potassium ATPase on the basolateral membrane removes three sodium ions from the cell and allows two potassium ions to enter. This results in the net removal of sodium and one positive charge from the cell interior, producing a low intracellular sodium concentration and a negative electrical potential inside the cell relative to both the lumen and the extracellular space. This electrochemical gradient favors entry of sodium from the lumen into

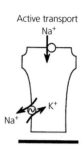

Figure 7.5 Active transport requires production of energy to move solute across the mucosa. *Primary active transport* involves pumps that directly couple energy creation from hydrolysis of ATP to movement of solute (e.g., sodium–potassium ATPase on basolateral membrane). The ion gradients produced by active transport can power *secondary active transport* at the apical membrane (e.g., glucose–sodium cotransport).

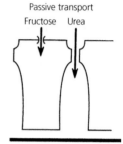

Figure 7.6 Passive transport involves passage of solute down its concentration through carriers (transcellular pathway) or through tight junctions (paracellular pathway).

the cell, and this thermodynamically "downhill" entry can be coupled to "uphill" transport of other solutes (such as glucose and amino acids) against their concentration gradients by proteins in the apical membrane (nutrient-linked cotransport). The sodium gradient can also power Na–H exchange across the apical membrane.

Passive transport refers to movement of solute down its electrochemical gradient (Figure 7.6) [1]. It is subject to differences in solute concentration and electrical potential between the lumen and plasma. In addition, passive transport depends on the permeability of the epithelium, which can be modulated by the opening of ion channels or the presence of proteins that facilitate diffusion or by the selective permeability of tight junctions.

Solvent drag (convective transport) occurs when rapid water transport entrains solute entry through paracellular pathways (Figure 7.7) [1]. In order to maintain osmotic equilibrium, water rushes through relatively leaky tight junctions in response to translocation of solute into the basolateral space. This flow of water entrains additional solute from the lumen. Since it depends on large absorptive fluxes of water through leaky tight junctions, solvent drag is quantitatively important only in the upper small intestine (duodenum and jejunum) where the epithelium is leakiest.

Intestinal absorption also is modified by the presence of luminal diffusion barriers. An unstirred water layer covers the apical membrane of the enterocyte and impedes the diffusion of molecules from the bulk solution in the lumen to the apical membrane where transport mechanisms can translocate the molecule

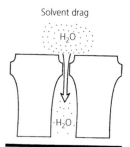

Figure 7.7 Solvent drag involves entrainment of solute in the stream of water passing through the tight junctions. It can only occur in the duodenum and jejunum where tight junctions are loose enough to produce large paracellular water fluxes.

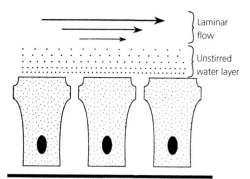

Figure 7.8 Fluid flow through the lumen and mixing of contents are optimal in the center of the lumen and decrease at the mucosal surface where water movement is very slow, producing an "unstirred water layer" that can serve as a diffusion barrier for large molecular arrays like mixed micelles.

into the enterocyte (Figure 7.8) [1]. Recent evidence suggests that this layer may be thinner than previously estimated but still thick enough to modulate the transport of some substances.

Water transport

As mentioned previously, water transport is thought to be secondary to solute transport [5]. The details of that coupling are not yet settled. The original concept was that active solute absorption produces a hypertonic compartment that draws in water, producing hydrostatic pressure that drives water into the extracellular compartment (standing-gradient model). Discovery of the basolateral spaces provided an anatomical basis for this theory. Some experimental observations, however, are inconsistent with the standing-gradient model, implying that the model is imperfect. Investigators have proposed that (i) sodium may be recycled across the basolateral membrane, secondarily drawing water across tight junctions; (ii) water entrapped in the apical sodium–glucose cotransporter enters the

Table 7.2 Luminal substances causing secretion.

Physiological agents
Guanylin (cGMP)
Bile acids (cAMP)
Long-chain fatty acids (cAMP)
Bacterial enterotoxins
Cholera toxin (cAMP)
Heat-labile *E. coli* toxin (cAMP)
Salmonella toxin (cAMP)
Campylobacter toxin (cAMP)
Heat-stable *E. coli* toxin (cGMP)
Yersinia toxin (cGMP)

intracellular space as the carrier engages in solute absorption (approximately 220–400 molecules of water per glucose molecule); and (iii) countercurrent exchange along the length of the villus results in a hypertonic villous tip that enhances water absorption. Each of these concepts has flaws too, and the standing-gradient model remains widely accepted as the standard model [5].

Water secretion in the intestine is thought to be mediated by chloride secretion across the apical membrane, largely by cystic fibrosis transmembrane regulator (CFTR), the main chloride channel in the apical membrane. This channel is inactive in persons with cystic fibrosis [4]. Chloride secretion draws sodium and water across tight junctions by generating electrical and osmotic gradients between the basolateral space and the lumen. Chloride secretion is regulated physiologically by guanylin, a peptide that is secreted into the lumen and interacts with the guanylin cyclase-C receptor on the apical surface of enterocytes to raise cyclic-GTP levels and open CFTR. This mechanism is co-opted by some bacterial toxins to produce diarrhea. Other mediators generating cyclic AMP or increasing intracellular calcium levels also trigger chloride and fluid secretion by the intestine (Table 7.2).

Sodium transport

Sodium–hydrogen exchange is mediated by a series of exchangers (NHE1–NHE10) located in mucosal cell membranes [8]. NHE1 is located in the basolateral membrane and is thought to be involved in regulation of intracellular pH and volume. NHE2 is located in the apical enterocyte membrane especially in

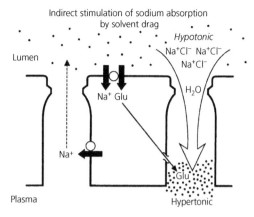

Figure 7.9 Glucose-stimulated sodium absorption in the jejunum likely involves solvent drag since most sodium that is absorbed transcellularly leaks back into the lumen through the paracellular pathway.

the right colon. Its role in fluid and electrolyte transport in humans is uncertain. In animals, it is most active in newborns. NHE3 seems to be an important marker of adult absorptive cells. It localizes to the apical membrane and plays an important role in epithelial sodium absorption. In the jejunum, sodium–hydrogen exchange results in net absorption of sodium and in acidification of the brush border membrane. In the ileum and colon, sodium–hydrogen exchange is coupled with chloride–bicarbonate exchange and results in neutral sodium chloride absorption.

Nutrient-coupled sodium absorption is an important mechanism for sodium absorption. Each molecule of glucose is cotransported with two sodium ions across the apical membrane and then is transported into the basolateral space. In the jejunum, this enhances net sodium absorption, in part by enhancing solvent drag (Figure 7.9) [9]. (Much of the cotransported sodium must leak back into the lumen, since more than 2 mol of sodium would be absorbed by cotransport of normal daily glucose intake, far exceeding renal excretory capacity.) Nutrient-coupled sodium absorption also occurs with amino acids.

Electrogenic sodium absorption is mediated by a sodium channel (ENaC) and is common in the distal colon [1]. Because tight junctions in the distal colon are selectively permeable to chloride and are very tight, sodium does not diffuse back into the lumen well despite the highest plasma-to-lumen sodium gradient of the intestine.

Sodium secretion in the small intestine is a consequence of chloride secretion. Entry of negatively charged anions augments passive sodium permeation through tight junctions [1].

Potassium transport

Little is known about intestinal mechanisms of potassium absorption and secretion. About 85% of a potassium load is absorbed in the small bowel, perhaps by means of a potassium–hydrogen exchanger. Potassium secretion by the colon has been reported in patients with pseudo-obstruction; it appears to be active, but the precise mechanism is not known [10]. Potassium channels are known to exist in the intestine [4].

Anion transport

Chloride, bicarbonate, and short-chain fatty anions (SCFA) are the three anions of most importance to intestinal physiology.

As discussed previously, chloride secretion is mediated by chloride channels on the apical membrane, mainly CFTR, and also by a lower-capacity channel, ClC-2 [4]. Chloride for secretion enters the enterocyte from the basolateral side via a Na–K–2Cl cotransporter (NKCC1) [11]. The activity of this cotransporter is coordinated with that of the apical chloride channels to maintain cell volume and integrity during active secretion.

Chloride is absorbed by two different mechanisms: (i) chloride–bicarbonate exchange in the ileum and colon (either coupled to NHE3 or independent) and (ii) passive permeation across tight junctions. Transport in the jejunum is mainly passive across leaky tight junctions in response to electrochemical gradients. Elsewhere in the intestine and colon, chloride absorption occurs via chloride–bicarbonate exchange mediated by the chloride–bicarbonate exchangers, SLC26A3 and SLC26A6 [12].

SLC26A3, originally called "downregulated in colonic adenoma," is a product of a large family of genes that is conserved in bacteria, plants, and animals. The proteins encoded by these genes are responsible for transport of chloride, sulfate, hydroxyl ion, bicarbonate, and oxalate, among other anions [12]. SLC26A3 is mutated in patients with congenital chloride diarrhea; absence of the transporter results in poor chloride absorption and systemic alkalosis beginning in infancy. SLC26A3 exchangers are functionally coupled with NHE3 exchangers to produce neutral sodium chloride absorption in the ileum and colon. The coupling seems to involve intracellular pH: bicarbonate secretion in exchange for chloride absorption via SLC26A3 acidifies the cell and stimulates compensatory hydrogen ion secretion by NHE3. Activation of SLC26A3 can result in net bicarbonate secretion if CFTR is open and allows chloride to reenter the lumen. This process depends on intracellular generation of bicarbonate by CA (Carbonic Anhydrase).

SLC26A6 appears to have similar functions to SLC26A3 in several species; its effect on chloride and bicarbonate transport in humans is less well understood. It does seem to be an important oxalate transporter in humans, leading to oxalate secretion in exchange for chloride [12].

SCFA are transported by products of the SLC16 gene family, monocarboxylate transporters and sodium-coupled monocarboxylate transporters [12]. On the apical surface, these transport proteins work as cotransporters for SCFA with either hydrogen ions or sodium ions accompanying SCFA into the cells. On the basolateral membrane, other members of this transporter family work as cotransporters to allow SCFA to exit the enterocyte.

Regional transport properties of the intestine

Transport in the duodenum and jejunum

The leakiest tight junctions in the bowel are in the proximal intestine. This makes osmotic equilibration quite rapid and water fluxes large. Solvent drag is an important mechanism for solute absorption in this part of the intestine. Transmembrane cation transport occurs by means of nutrient-linked cotransport and apical Na–H exchange. Because the tight junctions are leaky and cation selective, sodium ions cannot accumulate on the basolateral side of the enterocyte and diffuse back into the lumen, largely dissipating the electrical potential difference between the lumen and the extracellular space. This results in limited passive loss of potassium from the plasma. Chloride movement is also passive, but since the tight junctions are cation selective, chloride losses are limited. Bicarbonate transport is due to apical Na–H exchange that results in disappearance of bicarbonate from the lumen through reaction with secreted hydrogen ion; bicarbonate is regenerated within the enterocyte as hydrogen ions are produced by CA. A chloride secretory mechanism is present and can be activated in various situations (e.g., cholera toxin or other bacterial toxins). This portion of the bowel is designed to bring chyme into osmotic equilibrium. It is capable of absorbing most nutrients and much of the water and salt entering the intestine (Figure 7.10).

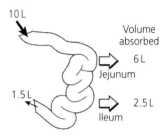

Figure 7.10 The bulk of water absorption occurs in the jejunum and ileum due to vigorous nutrient and sodium absorption in these regions of the intestine. Adapted from Reference [13]. Reproduced with permission of Elsevier.

Transport in the ileum

Ileal tight junctions are tighter than those of the jejunum, and thus, solvent drag plays a much smaller role in ileal solute transport. Most water transport is in response to solute movement due to neutral NaCl absorption (by means of paired Na–H and Cl–bicarbonate exchange) and residual Na–nutrient cotransport. Because the membrane is tighter, luminal potential difference is somewhat more negative (as compared to the basolateral side of the enterocyte) than in the jejunum, and passive potassium losses can occur. Chloride secretion can occur in the ileum and is triggered by similar agents as in the jejunum.

This portion of the intestine is well adapted to absorb salt, water, and residual nutrients from isotonic luminal contents. Acting together, the jejunum and ileum normally absorb 90% of the nearly 10 l of luminal contents passing the ligament of Treitz each day (Figure 7.10).

Transport in the colon

Transport across the colonic mucosa varies regionally. The tight junctions of the right colon are tighter than those of the ileum, and the tight junctions of the left colon are the tightest, maintaining the largest potential differences and chemical gradients of the entire intestine. The tight junctions are anion and not cation selective like those of the rest of the intestine. This limits the passive loss of sodium and potassium from the extracellular space that would occur with a large lumen-negative potential difference, and therefore, large concentration differences can develop across the mucosa (i.e., luminal sodium concentrations can be <10 mmol/l). Sodium transport occurs by neutral sodium chloride absorption (paired Na–H and Cl–bicarbonate exchange) and by electrogenic sodium absorption (chloride selectivity and the lumen-negative potential difference favor passive chloride absorption along with sodium). Nutrient–sodium cotransport does not occur in the colon, but several mechanisms are thought to facilitate absorption of short-chain fatty acids, products of bacterial carbohydrate fermentation. The colon is adapted to extract almost all of the sodium and most water from luminal contents (Figure 7.11). This is facilitated by the slow transit of luminal contents through the colon.

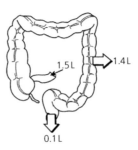

Figure 7.11 Colonic absorption removes almost all remaining water from the lumen as sodium is reduced to very low levels (~10 mmol/l). Adapted from [13]. Reproduced with permission of Elsevier.

Regulation of transport

A number of different regulators are known to affect intestinal transport under experimental conditions; however, the physiological regulation of transport is not clearly understood. It is likely that an interplay of luminal, humoral, neural, and immunological factors is involved. These extracellular signals cause biochemical changes within enterocytes that regulate transport processes.

Many different substances on the luminal side of the mucosa can affect intestinal transport (Table 7.2). Guanylin, a peptide secreted into the lumen, can increase chloride secretion. The extent to which this occurs physiologically and whether other luminal peptides alter absorption are uncertain. Other components of chyme, such as bile acids, can affect transport as well. In pathologic states, bacterial toxins (e.g., cholera toxin, *Escherichia coli* toxin) can reduce absorption and increase secretion by interacting with receptors on the apical enterocyte surface [1].

A rich collection of basolateral mediators potentially may regulate intestinal transport (Table 7.3). Steroid hormones, such as mineralocorticoids and glucocorticoids, can alter intestinal transport. Neurotransmitters, such as ACh and norepinephrine, also can affect transport. Peptides released from endocrine and immune cells and neurons also may be involved. Other agents, such as prostaglandins, histamine, and serotonin, released by cells in the submucosa also could alter intestinal transport.

These extracellular regulators alter transport by interacting with receptors on the basolateral cell membrane or in the nucleus. Intracellular mediators of their effects include the AC (G-protein) system, PKA, PLC, diacylglycerol, inositol triphosphate, calcium, and the guanylate-cyclase system. These mediators act by altering the activity of transport proteins and the properties of tight junctions.

Table 7.3 Endogenous agents that can alter intestinal transport from the basolateral surface.

Absorbagogues	Secretagogues
Aldosterone	Prostaglandins, leukotrienes
Alpha-adrenergic agonists	Vasoactive intestinal polypeptide, peptide-histidine isoleucine
Enkephalins	Secretin
SST	Substance P
Angiotensin	Neurotensin
Neuropeptide Y	ACh
Prolactin	Serotonin
Glucocorticoids	Histamine

Multiple choice questions

1 As regards tight junctions in the small intestine, which one of the following statements is *false*?

   A Tight junctions divide the apical domain of the basement membrane from the basolateral domain.

   B Tight junctions are more permeable to sodium ions than to chloride ions.

   C Tight junctions entirely prevent permeation of sodium ions from the basolateral space to the lumen.

   D Tight junction permeability is regulated.

   E Tight junctions are part of the apical junction complex that binds epithelial cells together.

2 As regards water transport across the gastrointestinal mucosa, which one of the following statements is *true*?

   A Water absorption is entirely due to active transport of sodium.

   B Water transport is entirely via transcellular mechanisms.

   C Water secretion may be mediated by chloride secretion.

   D Water transport in the jejunum occurs exclusively via aquaporins.

   E Water secretion is a result of the lumen-positive potential difference.

3 Which of the following regulatory substances causes chloride secretion in the small intestine from the luminal (apical) side of the enterocyte?

   A Guanylin

   B Acetylcholine

   C Serotonin

   D Epinephrine

   E Somatostatin

4 ONE BEST ANSWER: Na^+-dependent transport is responsible for the absorption of the following EXCEPT:

   A Amino acids

   B Fatty acids

   C Glucose

   D Galactose

References

1 Venkatasubramanian, J., Rao, M.C., and Sellin, J.H. (2010) Intestinal electrolyte absorption and secretion, in *Sleisenger & Fordtran's Gastrointestinal and Liver Disease*, 9th edn (eds M. Feldman, L. Friedman, and L.J. Brandt), Saunders Elsevier, Philadelphia, pp. 1675–1694.

2 Madara, J.L. and Trier, J.S. (1994) Functional morphology of the mucosa of the small intestine, in *Physiology of the Gastrointestinal Tract*, 3rd edn (eds L.R. Johnson, D.H. Alpers, J. Christensen E.D. Jacobson, and J.H. Walsh), Raven Press, New York.

3 Ortega, B. and Welling, P.A. (2012) Molecular mechanisms of protein sorting in polarized epithelial cells, in *Physiology of the Gastrointestinal Tract*, 5th edn (eds L.R. Johnson, F.K. Ghishan, J.D. Kaunitz *et al.*), Academic Press Elsevier, London, pp. 1559–1581.

4 Cuppoletti, J. and Malinowska, D.H. (2012) Ion channels of the epithelia of the gastrointestinal tract, in *Physiology of the Gastrointestinal Tract*, 5th edn (eds L.R. Johnson, F.K. Ghishan, J.D. Kaunitz *et al.*), Academic Press Elsevier, London, pp. 1863–1876.

5 Thiagarajah, J.R. and Verkman, A.S. (2012) Water transport in the gastrointestinal tract, in *Physiology of the Gastrointestinal Tract*, 5th edn (eds L.R. Johnson, F.K. Ghishan, J.D. Kaunitz JD *et al.*), Academic Press Elsevier, London, pp. 1757–1780.

6 Beaulieu, J.F. and Menard, D. (2012) Isolation, characterization, and culture of normal human intestinal crypt and villus cells. *Methods in Molecular Biology*, **806**, 157–173.

7 Ma, T.Y., Anderson, J.M. and Turner, J.R. (2012) Tight junctions and the intestinal barrier, in *Physiology of the Gastrointestinal Tract*, 5th edn (eds L.R. Johnson, F.K. Ghishan, J.D. Kaunitz *et al.*), Academic Press Elsevier, London, pp. 1043–1088.

8 Kiela, P.R. and Ghishan, F.K. (2012) Na^+/H^+ exchange in mammalian digestive tract, in *Physiology of the Gastrointestinal Tract*, 5th edn (eds L.R. Johnson, F.K. Ghishan, J.D. Kaunitz *et al.*), Academic Press Elsevier, London, pp. 1781–1818.

9 Schiller, L.R., Santa Ana, C.A., Porter, J. and Fordtran, J.S. (1997) Glucose-stimulated sodium transport by the human intestine during experimental cholera. *Gastroenterology*, **112**, 1529–1535.

10 Van Dinter, T.G. Jr., Fuerst, F.C., Richardson, C.T. *et al.* (2005) Stimulated active potassium secretion in a patient with colonic pseudo-obstruction: a new mechanism of secretory diarrhea. *Gastroenterology*, **129**, 1268–1273.

11 Haas, M. and Forbush, B. 3rd. (2000) The Na-K-Cl cotransporter of secretory epithelia. *Annual Review of Physiology*, **62**, 515–534.

12 Gill, R.K., Alrefai, W.A., Borthakur, A. and Dudeja, P.K. (2012) Intestinal anion absorption, in *Physiology of the Gastrointestinal Tract*, 5th edn (eds L.R. Johnson, F.K. Ghishan, J.D. Kaunitz *et al.*), Academic Press Elsevier, London, pp. 1819–1847.

13 Schiller, L.R. (2010) Chronic diarrhea, in *GI/Liver Secrets Plus*, 4th edn (ed P.R. McNally), Mosby Elsevier, Philadelphia, pp. 386–395.

Answers

1 C
2 C
3 A
4 B

CHAPTER 8

Absorption of nutrients

Lawrence R. Schiller

Dallas Campus, Texas A&M College of Medicine, Dallas, TX, USA
Digestive Health Associates of Texas, Dallas, TX, USA
Baylor University Medical Center, Dallas, TX, USA

Introduction

The fundamental function of the gut is to absorb nutrients. Alimentary tracts evolved in multicellular animals as the increasing complexity of body design meant that all tissues were no longer in contact with the surrounding environment. This necessitated the uptake of structural and energy-producing molecules by an absorptive epithelium and the distribution of these molecules throughout the body by the circulatory system. The mechanisms by which the absorptive epithelium transports nutrients evolved early in evolution and have been maintained intact in most existing phyla.

Humans are heterotrophs and must eat organic molecules synthesized by other living cells in order to survive. Many of the organic molecules that we eat are in the form of *polymers*, long chains of simpler compounds. For instance, starches are composed of long chains of sugars, and proteins are composed of chains of amino acids. Polymers could be absorbed intact (and to a limited extent are) by endocytosis, but the capacity of such a system is limited and absorption of intact polymers might induce allergic reactions. The paradigm employed by the human intestine is to digest polymers into simpler compounds that are moved across the epithelium by means of high-capacity transport pathways. These mechanisms allow each of us to efficiently absorb approximately 400 g of carbohydrate, 100 g of fat, and 90 g of protein daily. Almost all ingested absorbable nutrients are absorbed by the intestine. In addition to these macronutrients, essential micronutrients, such as vitamins and minerals, are absorbed by the intestine.

The human small intestine is adapted structurally to provide a large surface area for absorption [1]. In addition, the small intestine is adapted functionally to mix ingested nutrients with digestive enzymes and to distribute luminal contents over the absorptive surface in order to allow sufficient time for nutrient absorption. This process is subject to regulation by the neurohumoral regulatory

Gastrointestinal Anatomy and Physiology: The Essentials, First Edition. Edited by John F. Reinus and Douglas Simon.
© 2014 John Wiley & Sons, Ltd. Published 2014 by John Wiley & Sons, Ltd.
www.wiley.com/go/reinus/gastro/anatomy

system of the gut (enteric nerves and hormones). The portion of the small intestine that is most important for nutrient absorption is the jejunum, where a leaky epithelium allows rapid absorption of water and salt, thus concentrating nutrients and increasing the concentration gradients that drive absorptive processes. The ileum duplicates many of the nutrient-absorptive processes of the jejunum (and thus can compensate to some extent for malabsorption in the jejunum) and, in addition, has specialized absorption mechanisms, for example, for vitamin B_{12}. The colon has a very limited ability to absorb nutrients and, in this context, functions mainly to take up short-chain fatty acids (SCFA) that are products of carbohydrate fermentation by colonic bacteria.

Absorption of nutrients is largely a process of overcoming the thermodynamic barriers to mixing oil and water. Oily lipid molecules must be suspended in aqueous chyme, made accessible to water-soluble enzymes, and transported through aqueous luminal contents to the lipid cell membrane, where they can enter the cell's interior. Water-soluble nutrients, like carbohydrates and proteins, must get through the lipid cell membrane barrier. Nature has solved these problems by supplying detergent-like amphiphiles (bile acids) to solubilize luminal lipids and transmembrane transport proteins to allow water-soluble molecules to pass through the cell membrane.

Lipid absorption

Dietary fats include triglycerides, phospholipids, and cholesterol. Triglycerides provide a rich source of calories; phospholipids and cholesterol are important components of cell membranes. Some of these lipids have polar components that can interact with water. Others are mainly nonpolar and interact best with other lipids. The chemical characteristics of the lipids determine how these molecules interact with water. Lipid molecules orient themselves so that their polar groups interact with water and their nonpolar parts interact with each other. Because of this, in the aqueous environment of the gut lumen, lipids may form liquid crystals with lipid bilayers or thicker micelles each with polar elements facing their aqueous surroundings and nonpolar elements facing their interiors. Nonpolar lipids can accumulate in the cores of micelles. These transient structures are the form in which dietary lipid exists in the intestine, especially after lipolysis begins and fat becomes emulsified with water (Table 8.1).

Triglycerides are the major dietary fat in the human diet. These molecules have a polar glycerol backbone to which three fatty acid molecules are esterified. Fat digestion involves hydrolyzing the triglyceride to free fatty acids and monoglyceride that can be taken up by cells. This process starts in the acid environment of the stomach [2]. Lingual lipase is secreted by serous (von Ebner) glands at the base of the tongue. This enzyme is most active at an acid pH and so it begins to work in the stomach. Gastric lipase is secreted from peptic (chief) cells that also

Table 8.1 Schemes for lipid digestion and absorption.

	Triglyceride	Phospholipid	Cholesterol
Oral	Lingual lipase		
Gastric	Acidic lipases: diacylglycerol, FA Lingual lipase Gastric lipase		
Small bowel lumen	Solubilization by bile acids Micelles and liquid crystals Alkaline lipases: monoglycerol, FA Pancreatic lipase, colipase	Solubilization by bile acids Micelles and liquid crystals Phospholipase A$_2$	Solubilization by bile acids Micelles and liquid crystals Cholesterol esterase
Apical membrane digestion	None	None	None
Transport into enterocyte	Diffusion Carriers (CD36)→FA-binding proteins	Diffusion ? carriers	NPC1L1→clathrin-coated pits for internalization
Intracellular processing	Resynthesis of triglyceride Packaging into chylomicrons	Re-esterification with FA Packaging into chylomicrons, other lipoproteins	Re-esterification with FA Packaging into chylomicrons, other lipoproteins
Export from enterocyte	Exocytosis of chylomicrons, release of other lipoproteins	Exocytosis of chylomicrons, release of other lipoproteins	Exocytosis of chylomicrons, release of other lipoproteins Secretion of sitosterol and some cholesterol across apical membrane by ABCG5/ABCG8

FA, fatty acid;
NPC1L1, Niemann–Pick C$_1$-like protein 1;
ABCG5, ABCG8, ATP-binding cassette (ABC) proteins G5 and G8.

secrete pepsin. Like lingual lipase, it also can function in an acidic environment in the presence of pepsin. Neither of these acidic lipases requires bile acid or colipase to work. Gastric lipase acts solely on triglyceride (not phospholipid or esterified cholesterol). Medium-chain fatty acids are preferentially released, and free fatty acid and diacylglycerol are the predominant products. Gastric lipase is especially important in newborns for the digestion of milk fat and is responsible for most of the residual lipolytic activity in patients with total pancreatic exocrine insufficiency (about 30% of normal [2]). Production of free fatty acid and diacyl-glycerol in the stomach assists with emulsification of dietary lipid since these digestion products are more polar than unhydrolyzed triglyceride.

Chyme entering the intestine is alkalinized by bicarbonate-rich secretions from the pancreas. Lipid droplets interact with colipase and the alkaline lipases produced by the pancreas, such as pancreatic lipase and phospholipase A_2. Colipase binds to the lipid–water interface of the lipid droplet and to pancreatic lipase and facilitates the lipolytic activity of pancreatic lipase, which produces free fatty acids and monoglyceride that interact with bile acids, phospholipids, and cholesterol to form mixed micelles and liquid crystalline vesicles. These structures allow the reaction products to more efficiently cross the unstirred water layer that separates the brush border of the mucosa from the bulk phase of luminal fluid and release fatty acids and monoglyceride at the cell membrane.

The products of triglyceride digestion then are transported through the cell membrane into the enterocyte. Fatty acid translocase CD36 appears to play an important role in this process. Fatty acid-binding proteins chaperone potentially toxic free fatty acids from the cell membrane to the endoplasmic reticulum (ER) for further processing [3, 4]. Once fatty acid and monoglyceride reach the ER, triglyceride is resynthesized. Apolipoproteins and other lipids are added in the Golgi apparatus to form chylomicrons that are released by exocytosis into the basolateral space for distribution via lymphatics to the rest of the body.

Phospholipid is digested in the small intestine by pancreatic phospholipase A_2. This enzyme is secreted as a proenzyme, is activated by trypsin, and requires bile salt for its activity. The hydrolytic products are then taken up by the mucosa in a process that is thought to be similar to that for the products of triglyceride digestion. Phospholipids can be resynthesized and exported in chylomicrons or very-low-density lipoproteins or further degraded and then secreted into portal blood.

Most ingested cholesterol is not esterified, and the cholesterol that is esterified to fatty acid must be hydrolyzed before absorption. This is accom-plished by a pancreatic enzyme, cholesterol esterase. Cholesterol uptake by the cell membrane is specific, is energy dependent, and is facilitated by Niemann–Pick C_1-like protein 1 (NPC1L1), which is expressed in the apical brush border membrane [5]. NPC1L1 helps to transport cholesterol across the cell mem-brane and binds to adaptor protein 2 (AP2) and to clathrin to form a small vesicle analogous to a coated pit that shuttles cholesterol into the interior of the cell. This process can be inhibited by milligram amounts of ezetimibe, an inhibitor of the interaction of NPC1L1, cholesterol, and AP2–clathrin. Cycling of NPC1L1 seems to be regulated by intracellular cholesterol levels [5]. Cholesterol is exported from the basolateral surface of the enterocyte in chylomicrons and other lipoprotein particles.

Cholesterol and plant sterols also can be secreted into the lumen across the apical membrane of the enterocyte. This plays an important role in reducing absorption of sitosterol, a potentially toxic plant sterol, and may modulate net cholesterol absorption [6]. Recent work has identified ATP-binding cassette (ABC) proteins, ABCG5 and ABCG8, as transporters for cholesterol and sitosterol [3]. These proteins may also be responsible for biliary cholesterol excretion.

Protein absorption

Humans rely on ingested protein to supply essential amino acids: valine, leucine, isoleucine, phenylalanine, tryptophan, tyrosine, methionine, lysine, and histidine. The other amino acids used to make human proteins can be synthesized from other compounds and also can be absorbed from the diet. Approximately 70–100 g of protein is contained in the average daily diet. Amino acids are used to create structural proteins but can be metabolized to produce energy. In order to be used for structural purposes and not as fuel, sufficient nonprotein calories must be available for metabolism.

The scheme for protein digestion and absorption is hydrolysis of the linear polymer into amino acids and di- and tripeptides in the aqueous luminal environment and transport of these products across the cell membrane [7]. Since proteins are water soluble, soluble luminal enzymes can interact with dietary proteins without encountering a phase boundary. The variety of potential amino acid combinations makes several types of proteolytic enzymes necessary. Mucosal transport also must be tailored to the different chemical characteristics of biologically important amino acids. Thus, several distinct transporters are needed.

Protein digestion begins in the acid environment of the stomach with pepsin and another gastric protease, chymosin (rennin). Pepsin is synthesized and secreted by chief cells in the stomach as pepsinogen. This molecule is activated to pepsin by acid hydrolysis (pH < 4) in the stomach and is inactivated at higher pH levels (inhibited at pH > 5.5, denatured at pH > 7.2). It attacks a broad range of peptide bonds and releases peptides and amino acids in the stomach that stimulate gastrin release by the antrum until the protein load is emptied from the stomach. Chymosin (rennin) is more prominent in the neonatal period and is particularly active in cleaving milk proteins (hence its use to curdle milk for cheese making).

Protein digestion continues in the duodenum where acid chyme stimulates release of secretin, which causes pancreatic bicarbonate secretion. Protein and fat in chyme also stimulate release of cholecystokinin (CCK) that stimulates pancreatic enzyme secretion. Pancreatic proteases are secreted as proenzymes that are activated in the lumen of the duodenum by enterokinase, a brush border enzyme. Trypsin activated by enterokinase can activate the other enzymes. These enzymes are only active at near-neutral or alkaline luminal acidity; thus, pancreatic bicarbonate secretion is essential to their function. By convention, pancreatic pro-teases are classified as endopeptidases (e.g., trypsin, chymotrypsin, elastase) that cleave interior peptide bonds and exopeptidases (e.g., carboxypeptidases A and B) that hydrolyze amino acids from the ends of peptide chains. Endopeptidases target specific peptide bonds in the protein chain. Trypsin cleaves the peptide chain next to lysine and arginine; chymotrypsin attacks the bond next to tyrosine, phenylal-anine, and tryptophan; elastase hydrolyzes the chain next to alanine, leucine, glycine, valine, and isoleucine. The end result of this process is a mix of peptides containing on average six to eight amino acids. Secretion of pancreatic enzymes is stimulated by pancreatic nerves and by CCK released by the duodenal mucosa and is inhibited by several peptide hormones, including pancreatic polypeptide and somatostatin (SST), and by feedback from the duodenal mucosa.

The products of intraluminal digestion diffuse to the brush border. There, more than a dozen different membrane-bound endopeptidases, aminopepti-dases, carboxypeptidases, and dipeptidases complete digestion of polypeptides to amino acids and di- and tripeptides that can be transported across the cell membrane [7]. Quantitatively, more amino acids may be taken up as di- and tripeptides than as free amino acids. Transport of free amino acids is handled by several discrete systems of transporters that have specific chemical selectivity. Several of these systems are energized by the inwardly directed sodium gra-dient maintained by the basolateral Na^+–K^+-ATPase pump. Intact dipeptides and tripeptides are transported into the enterocyte by different mechanisms than free amino acids; intracellular peptidases cleave di- and tripeptides to free amino acids. Absorption of these intact peptides is energized by an inwardly directed H^+ gradient produced by Na^+–H^+ exchange across the brush border. Absorbed amino acids are metabolized, used for enterocyte protein synthesis, or secreted into the blood by enterocytes. At least six different transport systems are involved with the export of amino acids from enterocytes into the blood. There also are transporters in the basolateral membrane of the enterocyte that can import amino acids from the blood during fasting.

There is evidence that small amounts of intact proteins and peptides can be absorbed by pinocytosis [8]. This may be important immunologically but is of such limited capacity that it does not seem to be important nutritionally. Whether substantial amounts of protein, peptides, or amino acids traverse the paracellular pathway in humans is unknown (but seems unlikely given the permeability characteristics of the tight junctions) (Table 8.2).

Carbohydrate absorption

Carbohydrates comprise the largest source of calories in the human diet [9]. Dietary carbohydrate molecules are of three kinds: monosaccharides, such as glucose and fructose; oligosaccharides, mainly sucrose and lactose; and polysaccharides,

Table 8.2 Schemes for protein digestion and absorption.

	Amino acids	Di- and tripeptides	Polypeptides and proteins
Oral	None	None	None
Gastric	None	None	Pepsin, chymosin (rennin): release of smaller peptides, amino acids

Small bowel lumen	None	Minimal	Endopeptidases
			  Trypsin
			  Chymotrypsin
			  Elastase
			Exopeptidases
			  Carboxypeptidase A
			  Carboxypeptidase B

Apical membrane digestion	None	Some digestion to amino acids, most di- and tripeptides are taken up intact	Further digestion of peptide fragments by multiple membrane-bound endopeptidases, aminopeptidases, carboxypeptidases, and dipeptidases
Transport into enterocyte	Several discrete and chemically selective carrier systems, some involving sodium cotransport	Several discrete carrier systems, some involving sodium cotransport	Minimal uptake of intact peptides by pinocytosis, mainly for immunological purposes
Intracellular processing	Resynthesis of peptides	Intracellular di- and tripeptidases produce free amino acids which are available for resynthesis of peptides or export	Degradation of peptides
Export from enterocyte	Basolateral amino acid transport systems (~90%)	Some di- and tripeptides secreted intact (~10%)	Some newly synthesized protein may be secreted

including starch, glycogen, and fiber (e.g., cellulose, gums, pectins). Monosaccharides are absorbed by selective mechanisms that preferentially transport specific sugars across the enterocyte cell membrane. Disaccharides, such as sucrose and lactose, are cleaved by specific disaccharidases in the brush border, and the resulting monosaccharides are transported across the cell membrane. Polymeric carbohydrates, such as starch, must undergo intraluminal digestion before brush border processing and transport. Humans lack enzymes to digest some polymeric carbohydrate ("dietary fiber") and these can't be absorbed.

More than half of dietary carbohydrate intake is in the form of starch, a storage form of glucose in plants. Starch molecules are polymers composed of glucose molecules in long chains (amylose) and branched forms (amylopectin). Salivary amylase begins the process of starch digestion in the mouth. Like pancreatic amylase, with which it has significant homology, it attacks internal α-1,4 glucose bonds and cleaves starch into maltotriose (trimer), maltose (dimer), and α-limit dextrins (5–10 glucose units including an α-1,6 branch point). Free glucose molecules are not produced by amylase. These cleavage products are sweet and contribute to the taste of many carbohydrates. Salivary amylase is inactivated by gastric acid, but starch digestion continues with pancreatic amylase in the duodenum. Amylase is secreted by the pancreas in an active form. (Starch is not part of the human body and so autodigestion is not a risk.) The activity of pancreatic amylase depends on calcium and chloride ions in the duodenum.

The oligosaccharides produced by amylase and ingested oligosaccharides are further digested by four brush border enzymes: sucrase–isomaltase, lactase–phlorizin hydrolase, glucoamylase, and trehalase. Examples of substrates for these enzymes are sucrose (cane sugar), lactose (milk sugar), maltotriose and maltose, and trehalose (a sugar found in some fungi), respectively. These enzymes release glucose, galactose, and fructose in high concentration adjacent to the brush border where they can be transported into the cell interior.

The transporter for glucose has been studied extensively [9]. Glucose is absorbed rapidly across the brush border by a process that is saturable, that is specific for D-glucose, and that requires energy. The energy is provided by the Na$^+$–K$^+$-ATPase located on the basolateral membrane of the enterocyte. This pump removes Na$^+$ from the cell interior, creating an electrochemical gradient for sodium entry into the cell. By coupling glucose entry to sodium entry across the apical (brush border) membrane, glucose can be absorbed against its concentration gradient. The agent that couples the entry of these two substances is the Na$^+$/glucose cotransporter (SGLT1), a protein that spans the apical membrane 14 times. SGLT1 is expressed in the upper third of the villus. Galactose also can be transported with sodium by the same cotransporter and with the same kinetics. This protein transports two Na$^+$ ions for each sugar molecule. An elaborate mechanism has been postulated for the action of this cotransporter, somewhat analogous to an airlock on a spacecraft [9]. Sodium binds first to the luminal side of a cleft formed by the transporter, opening a luminal-side gate and increasing its affinity for binding sugar. The sugar-2-Na$^+$-cotransporter complex then isomerizes so that the cleft geometry changes, the luminal gate closes, and the intracellular gate opens. The sodium and sugar now face the interior of the cell. The sugar dissociates and enters the cytoplasm, and then, the sodium is released into the cell. The transporter then recycles.

Fructose crosses the brush border by facilitated diffusion via a separate apical transport protein, GLUT5. Entry of this sugar can be as rapid as that of glucose or galactose but occurs down the fructose concentration gradient and is sodium independent. The capacity for fructose absorption is limited due to limited expression of GLUT5 and can be overwhelmed by high fructose intake, resulting in fructose malabsorption [10].

Glucose, galactose, and fructose exit from the enterocyte across its basolateral membrane by means of another sugar transporter, GLUT2. Transport occurs by facilitated diffusion and is sodium independent [9].

Transcellular transport by proteins with specific binding requirements accounts for the selectivity of intestinal carbohydrate absorption. Although it has been hypothesized that paracellular sugar transport can account for a substantial portion of mucosal sugar absorption, such a process would not be stereoselective, and careful studies in humans show that substantial paracellular glucose transport is unlikely to occur [11, 12].

Another recent insight concerns the fate of sodium cotransported with sugar. If 300 g (1.67 mol) of glucose and galactose are absorbed each day by cotransport, a total of 3.34 mol (76.8 g) of sodium would be cotransported daily. This is much more sodium than could possibly be excreted by the kidneys each day. In fact, because chloride permeability in the jejunum is limited as compared to sodium, most sodium that is transported to the basolateral side of the enterocyte by cotransport diffuses back to the lumen through the paracellular pathway (tight junction) because of the electrochemical gradient produced by sodium absorption [13]. This recycling of sodium means that glucose absorption is never limited by luminal sodium availability *in vivo* and can proceed to completion by the time that chyme reaches the ileum.

Although the colon lacks mucosal mechanisms for disaccharide digestion and monosaccharide uptake, carbohydrate entering the colon can be salvaged by bacterial fermentation and absorption of fermentation products, such as SCFA [14]. The amount of carbohydrate delivered to the colon depends upon diet. Indigestible carbohydrate including dietary fiber and incompletely absorbed sugars and sugar alcohols, such as fructose, oligosaccharides, and sorbitol, may be an appreciable part of overall dietary content. It has been estimated on the basis of breath hydrogen studies that about 10% of ingested wheat starch enters the colon, largely due to difficulty in digesting gluten on the surface of the wheat starch granule [15].

Once carbohydrate enters the colon, the fecal flora ferments carbohydrate into SCFA, hydrogen gas and carbon dioxide gas. Based on studies with ingested lactulose, the colonic flora can metabolize approximately 80 g of lactulose per day [16]. SCFA are absorbed by nonionic diffusion of the protonated anion across the apical membrane, by cotransport with sodium or hydrogen or by SCFA–bicarbonate exchange [17]. SCFA–H$^+$ cotransport is mediated by monocarboxylate transporter-1 (MCT1) in the apical membrane. The activity of this transporter is increased by SST, leptin, butyrate, and pectin and decreased by enteropathogenic

Escherichia coli and inflammation. SCFA–Na$^+$ cotransport is thought to be mediated by sodium-coupled monocarboxylate transporter 1 in the apical membrane.

Under ordinary conditions, carbohydrate salvage via fermentation to SCFA makes only a minor contribution to energy supplies in humans. When malabsorption occurs (as with pancreatic exocrine insufficiency), as much as 10% of energy requirements may be met by fermentation and colonic absorption of SCFA [18]. Absorbed SCFA also may mediate metabolic effects on adipose tissue and pancreatic islets that tend to reduce obesity and improve glucose tolerance by actions on free fatty acid receptors (FFAR2 and FFAR3) [14] (Table 8.3).

Mineral absorption

Calcium

Calcium is essential to growth and development of the skeleton, muscle activity, and intracellular signaling [19]. An average 70-kg adult contains 1 kg of calcium, 99% of which is in bones and teeth. Calcium concentration in extracellular fluid is regulated tightly by the body and is kept within narrow limits. Intracellular calcium concentration is very low, allowing calcium entry into cells to be used as a major signaling mechanism for cell function. Dietary calcium intake ranges from 400 to 1000 mg daily, and it is incompletely absorbed. Calculation of absorption is complicated by the fact that calcium also enters the intestinal lumen as part of intestinal and exocrine secretions; the part of this flux of calcium that is not absorbed is known as endogenous fecal calcium and represents a constitutive loss that must be offset by absorption. Calcium absorption is regulated by vitamin D in response to dietary availability and body needs.

Calcium is absorbed by both active and passive mechanisms. Calcium must be solubilized before absorption; this can be done by gastric acid, but acidification of the luminal fluid adjacent to the brush border in the jejunum by Na$^+$–H$^+$ exchange can be sufficient. Active calcium absorption occurs across the brush border membrane of enterocytes in the small intestine; presumably, calcium ions enter the cytoplasm by going through channels or by interacting with carriers. Calcium entry into the enterocyte occurs down an electrochemical gradient (the interior of the cell has a [Ca^{+2}] of 100 nM and has a more negative electrical potential than the lumen). Molecular studies point to transient receptor potential vanilloid (TRPV) 6 as the major channel involved in facilitated diffusion of calcium across the brush border [19]. The activity of this channel can be upregulated by vitamin D (see the succeeding text) and downregulated by increased intracellular calcium. Once across the brush border, calcium ions interact with a calcium-binding protein, calbindin-D$_{9k}$ (CBD$_{9k}$), that protects the cell from an abrupt influx of free calcium ions and transports calcium across the cell to the basolateral membrane. There, calcium is extruded from the cell against its electrochemical gradient by an energy-requiring Ca^{+2}-ATPase (PMCA1b) [19].

Table 8.3 Schemes for carbohydrate digestion and absorption.

	Monosaccharides	Oligosaccharides (2–10 sugar units)	Polysaccharides (digestible)	Polysaccharides (indigestible/poorly digestible)
Oral	None	None	Salivary amylase	None
Gastric	None	None	None	None
Small bowel lumen	None	None	Pancreatic amylase	None
Apical membrane digestion	None	Sucrase–isomaltase Lactase–phlorizin hydrolase Glucoamylase Trehalase	Further digestion of oligosaccharides by brush border enzymes listed to the left	None
Transport into enterocyte	SGLT1 (glucose, galactose; cotransport with sodium) GLUT5 (fructose; carrier-facilitated diffusion)	As monosaccharides only	None	None
Intracellular processing	None	None	None	None
Export from enterocyte	GLUT2 (facilitated diffusion for glucose, galactose, fructose)	None	None	None
Colonic processing	Fermentation by bacteria	Fermentation by bacteria	Fermentation by bacteria	Fermentation by bacteria to SCFA; absorption of SCFA by diffusion, SCFA–HCO$_3$ exchange, SCFA–Na$^+$ cotransport, SCFA–H$^+$ cotransport

SGLT1, Na$^+$–glucose cotransporter; GLUT5, GLUT2, glucose transporter 5, glucose transporter 2; SCFA, short-chain fatty acid.

Vitamin D seems to have effects on calcium entry and extrusion. TRPV6, CBD_{9k}, and PMCA1b are upregulated by $1,25(OH)_2$-vitamin D_3. Active transport by this mechanism is important at low calcium intakes, can be saturated, and is regulated by renal production of activated vitamin D. Passive mechanisms are quantitatively more important with high calcium intake. When calcium intake is >500 mg daily, active transport mechanisms are saturated, and passive calcium absorption accounts for almost all of the increase in calcium absorption. Passive mechanisms probably involve paracellular transport and permit absorption of approximately one-third of calcium intake once active mechanisms are saturated [20].

Magnesium

Magnesium is critical to the action of many enzymes, muscle and nerve function, DNA and RNA activity, and calcium and potassium homeostasis [19]. It is the fourth most common cation in the body (after sodium, potassium, and calcium). It is the most common intracellular divalent cation and most of the magnesium in the body is intracellular; circulating concentrations do not accurately reflect body stores. Magnesium intake often is marginal and, given its poor absorption by the intestine, may be insufficient for needs, especially under conditions of increased loss due to intestinal or renal disease.

Like calcium, magnesium is absorbed by both active and passive mechanisms, but fractional absorption of magnesium is much less than that of calcium once active mechanisms are saturated, probably because of lower mucosal permeability [21]. The active mechanism is thought to be transcellular and involve facilitated diffusion across the apical membrane using a channel composed of a heterotetramer of TRPM6 and TRPM7 [19]. Extrusion across the basolateral membrane is thought to involve a sodium–magnesium exchanger or a magnesium pump, but experimental validation is lacking. Passive absorption likely occurs via the paracelluar (tight junction) pathway, but is not very efficient.

Unlike calcium, magnesium is more avidly absorbed in the ileum than in the jejunum. Vitamin D influences its absorption in the jejunum but not in the ileum. Even under the best of circumstances, magnesium absorption is incomplete; only 7% of a large magnesium load is absorbed in humans [21]. This allows magnesium salts to be used as osmotic laxatives.

Phosphate

Phosphorus is essential both as a structural element of the skeleton and as a key metabolic mediator [19]. Eighty-five percent of phosphate is in bone, 14% is intracellular, and only 1% is in extracellular fluids. Inside cells, it is the major storage form of chemical energy in the forms of ATP and creatine phosphate. About 800 mg of phosphate is ingested each day, mainly from dairy products, meat, and grains, and two-thirds is absorbed. Phosphate absorption is both active (sodium dependent) and passive (sodium independent). Vitamin D stimulates active absorption and is most important at lower luminal phosphate concentrations [22]. Passive mechanism predominates at higher luminal concentrations.

The mechanisms of phosphate absorption are still being studied. Entry into the enterocyte across the brush border is mediated by a type IIb sodium–phosphate (NaPi-IIb) cotransporter [19]. Three sodium ions enter the cell with each phosphate ion. Absorbed phosphate comingles with the cytosolic pool and can be exported across the basolateral membrane, likely by facilitated diffusion (the identity of the transporter is unconfirmed). Paracellular entry across tight junctions in the small intestine has been thought to be the main mechanism of passive (sodium-independent) absorption. This mechanism is relatively inefficient, however, allowing phosphate salts to be used as orally administered laxatives.

Trace elements

Iron

Iron is essential for distribution of oxygen to body tissues and is incorporated into hemoglobin and myoglobin. It participates in electron transfer as part of energy metabolism and cytochrome function. Iron also is toxic and its levels must be controlled precisely. Given that there is no efficient physiologic mechanism for iron excretion, regulation of absorption must be nearly perfect [23]. Approximately 1 mg of iron must be absorbed daily by men and up to 2 mg daily by women to maintain normal iron stores. Since absorption efficiency may be as low as 1–2%, intakes of up to 200 mg daily may be necessary to maintain homeostasis.

The duodenum is the major site of iron absorption. Ferric (Fe^{+3}) iron is insoluble and therefore must be reduced to the ferrous (Fe^{+2}) form to be absorbed. This can occur at the brush border of the duodenum where cytochrome b may work as a reductase. Dietary ascorbic acid also may play a role in this process. Inorganic ferrous iron is transported with hydrogen ion across the brush border membrane by divalent metal transporter 1 (DMT1). Then, Fe^{+2} either is transported to the basolateral membrane for export or is stored as ferritin within the enterocyte until it is needed elsewhere. Iron incorporated into heme (ingested hemoglobin or myoglobin) is taken up as intact heme probably by a transporter. Most is oxidized by heme oxygenase to ferrous iron; some may be transported across the basolateral membrane as intact heme.

In response to increased requirements (e.g., anemia, pregnancy), iron is exported from the hepatocyte at the basolateral membrane by ferroportin 1 (FPN1). Ferrous iron complexed with FPN1 is oxidized to the ferric form by a copper-containing iron-oxidase protein, hephaestin, for release and transport by transferrin.

Entry of iron into the body is tightly regulated [23]. A peptide made by the liver, hepcidin, is the main regulator of iron homeostasis. It is synthesized when iron stores are adequate and suppresses iron absorption in the gut and release of body iron stores. When more iron is needed, hepcidin levels drop, allowing movement of iron into the circulation. Hepcidin is regulated by physiologic signals reflective of hypoxia, inflammation, and body iron stores. Modulators of hepcidin release include hemojuvelin (HJV), HFE protein in conjunction with transferrin receptors 1 and 2 (TFR1/TFR2), and interleukin-6 (IL-6). HJV mediates the effects of bone morphogenetic protein 6 (BMP6); the concentration of this protein is proportional to body iron levels. Binding of BMP6 to HJV activates SMAD signaling, which ultimately increases hepcidin release and suppresses release of iron into the circulation [23]. HFE protein is an immunoglobulin-like molecule that associates with β2-microglobin and regulates the activity of TFR1 and TFR2. These receptors signal the cell to increase hepcidin production when there is sufficient circulating diferric transferrin. The common form of hereditary hemochromatosis involves a homozygous mutation (C282Y) of the *HFE* gene that interferes with this signaling, suppressing hepcidin release. Inflammation, mediated by the IL-6 receptor, also results in inhibition of hepcidin production.

Because iron may be stored as ferritin in the enterocyte, not all the iron that crosses the apical membrane is delivered to the circulation. In essence, the rate at which iron enters the circulation and the rate at which enterocytes are shed into the lumen compete to determine the net rate of iron absorption.

Copper

Copper is an essential nutrient that is absorbed by a process similar to that of iron [24]. Copper must be in its divalent form to be absorbed; like iron, a brush border reductase is involved in changing its valence. CTR1 is the apical membrane transporter for copper ions. Absorption is dose dependent; on average, about 50% of intake can be absorbed. Metallothionein is the intracellular-binding protein for copper, and ATP7A, a P-type ATPase, is the copper transporter in the basolateral membrane. (Menkes disease, a copper deficiency disorder, is due to failure to export copper into the circulation due to mutations in the *ATP7A* gene.) Ceruloplasmin, albumin, and amino acids are transporters for copper released into the circulation. Copper is removed from the circulation by the liver, and some is secreted into the bile by ATP7B, another copper transporter. (Both copies of the *ATP7B* gene are mutated in patients with Wilson's disease, who fail to excrete excess copper and accumulate copper systemically.) Copper secreted into the bile enters the duodenum where it can be reabsorbed along with dietary copper, and so a sort of enterohepatic copper circulation exists.

Copper absorption is saturable and is regulated in part by dietary copper load. Large amounts of ingested zinc interfere with copper absorption, but the mechanism of the interaction has not been thoroughly worked out. Competition for a transporter or altered regulation of copper metabolism could account for this finding.

Zinc

Zinc is another divalent cation that is absorbed both by an active, saturable process at low intraluminal concentrations and by a passive mechanism at higher concentrations. Luminal concentration from dietary intake rarely gets above the saturation threshold (1.8 mmol/l), so most dietary zinc is absorbed by the carrier-mediated, saturable route [24]. The apical membrane transporter is called Zip4, and its transcription is regulated by intracellular zinc levels. Mutations of both *Zip4* genes cause the autosomal recessive disease, acrodermatitis enteropathica, characterized by zinc deficiency. The disease can be treated by large doses of oral zinc.

Zinc, copper, and iron can interfere with each others' absorption. In part, this seems to be mediated by effects on metallothionein, but other interactions are possible. Zinc is transported out of the cell by the transporter ZnT-1 in the basolateral membrane [24].

Some zinc (up to 5 mg daily) is lost into the intestine as part of normal secretions [24]. Greater losses may occur with a variety of diarrheal diseases; supplementing zinc intake may be important in reducing the morbidity of these disorders.

Other trace elements

Less than 25% of dietary manganese is absorbed. It may utilize the same transport mechanisms as iron to cross the apical membrane (DMT1) and may use some of the same export mechanisms at the basolateral membrane, but this point is controversial [24]. Iodine and fluorine can be absorbed by the mechanisms used by chloride. In addition, iodinated amino acids can be absorbed as such by amino acid uptake mechanisms. Selenium and some forms of arsenic also may be taken up when bound to amino acids. Molybdenum, arsenic, boron, and vanadium are found in the diet largely bound to oxygen as ions analogous to sulfate or phosphate; they can be absorbed by the mechanisms used by sulfate or phosphate.

Vitamin absorption

Vitamins are essential micronutrients that cannot be synthesized by an organism [25]. Most function as required cofactors or coenzymes in the chemical reactions of normal metabolism. They also may have pharmacologic effects when taken in large amounts.

Vitamins may be characterized as either fat or water soluble and are absorbed in the same way as macronutrients that have similar properties. Like fat, esterified fat-soluble vitamins are hydrolyzed intraluminally and then transported across the apical enterocyte membrane. Water-soluble vitamins typically undergo intraluminal modification of extended side chains and then are transported across the apical membrane by carriers or endocytosis.

Vitamin D

In humans, vitamin D is perhaps more accurately thought of as a steroid hormone rather than as a vitamin. It is synthesized in skin exposed to sunlight and activated in the kidney, and so, we are not strictly dependent upon exogenous sources. Nevertheless, outside equatorial areas, endogenous vitamin D synthesis frequently is inadequate, particularly during the winter, and so, an exogenous source often is needed for health [26].

Vitamin D occurs in the diet as the free, unesterified sterols, cholecalciferol (vitamin D_3) and ergocalciferol (vitamin D_2). These may be absorbed like other lipids by passive diffusion, but carriers also may be involved. Bile acids are important to the digestion of dietary fat containing vitamin D. Most absorbed vitamin D is exported in chylomicrons and then transferred to vitamin D-binding protein in the circulation for distribution to the rest of the body. In the liver, vitamin D is converted to 25-hydroxyvitamin D, the metabolite measured to test vitamin D levels.

The active form of vitamin D, 1, 25-dihydroxyvitamin D_3, is produced in the kidney from 25-hydroxyvtamin D and interacts with a vitamin D receptor (VDR) in the nucleus of the enterocyte to regulate the expression of a number of different genes that modify calcium absorption [27]. These include genes that regulate production of TRPV5, TRPV6, calbindins, and PMCA1b. The net effect of these changes is to increase active calcium absorption by the enterocyte. VDR may have other effects, such as inducing enzymes that inactivate xenobiotic compounds and suppressing the activity of c-MYC, a proliferative factor in colon cancer.

Vitamin A

Vitamin A represents a family of biologically active retinoids, derived from dietary carotenoids, which are water-insoluble lipids. They are synthesized by plants and microorganisms and must be obtained from the diet [28]. Most dietary vitamin A precursors are esterified to long-chain fatty acids. These retinyl esters are hydrolyzed by pancreatic enzymes in the small intestine in the presence of bile acids and are thought to be taken up by a saturable, passive carrier-mediated mechanism [28]. They are then re-esterified to long-chain fatty acids and exported in chylomicrons. Carotenoids are absorbed by a passive, non-carrier-mediated mechanism and are converted to retinal by oxidation in the enterocyte. Retinal is further oxidized to retinoic acid or reduced to retinol. Retinyl esters are taken up by the liver and are then hydrolyzed and released as retinol coupled to serum retinol-binding protein for distribution to the body.

Folate

Folic or pteroylglutamic acid is composed of three covalently bonded parts: pteridine and para-aminobenzoic acid (together forming pteroic acid) and a single molecule of L-glutamic acid [29]. Polyglutamate folates consist of up to an additional six L-glutamic acid residues attached together by unique γ-glutamyl bonds in a long chain. Dietary folate consists of a mixture of free and polyglutamate forms. The extra glutamic acid residues have to be removed by hydrolysis prior to absorption. This occurs by means of folate hydrolase in the brush border of the jejunum. Free folic acid is then transported into the enterocyte by means of a saturable, carrier-mediated mechanism. Two different transport systems have been identified in the intestine: RFC and PCFT. When present in supraphysiological concentrations, folic acid also can be transported by a nonsaturable mechanism, but it is unclear whether this is transcellular or paracellular. At physiological doses, much of the folate traversing the enterocyte is reduced and methylated prior to release into the circulation.

Folate also is produced by bacteria in the colon. Most of this is in the absorbable monoglutamate form and can be absorbed by colonocytes via a carrier-mediated mechanism.

Cobalamin (B_{12})

Vitamin B_{12} is manufactured only by microorganisms but is essential to mammalian metabolism. Although bacteria in the colon can make B_{12}, it cannot be absorbed by the colon, and so, we depend on eating meat and dairy products for our supply of B_{12}. (It is not made in plants; strict vegans must supplement their diets with vitamin B_{12}.) The molecule is a large, complex structure consisting of a heme-like tetrapyrrole ring ("corrin") that contains cobalt instead of iron, attached to a nucleoside-like structure [29].

Dietary B_{12} is bound to dietary protein and is released by protein digestion in the stomach and upper intestine. In the stomach, two B_{12}-binding proteins, intrinsic factor and haptocorrin (R-protein, produced in the salivary glands), compete for B_{12}. Haptocorrin is better able to bind B_{12} at acid pH levels, and so in the stomach, most B_{12} binds to it. Haptocorrin is susceptible to digestion by pancreatic enzymes, and so, B_{12} is released in the upper intestine and then binds to intrinsic factor. The intrinsic factor–B_{12} complex then travels to the ileum where it is bound to a specific receptor, cubam, composed of cubilin which actually binds to intrinsic factor and amnionless, which is required for receptor-mediated endocytosis. Once the complex enters the cell, cobalamin then dissociates from intrinsic factor in lysosomes, is transported across the basolateral membrane by ATP-dependent MRP1, and binds to transcobalamin II, a B_{12}-binding protein in the basolateral space. The transcobalamin–B_{12} complex then enters the circulation to transport B_{12} throughout the body.

Thiamin

Thiamin is a water-soluble vitamin essential as a cofactor for many metabolic pathways. Most dietary thiamin is phosphorylated and must be hydrolyzed to free thiamine before absorption [29]. Two carriers, THTR-1 and THTR-2, shuttle thiamine across the apical surface of the enterocyte. Free thiamine exits across the basolateral membrane by means of an electroneutral, carrier-mediated mechanism.

Riboflavin

Like folate, riboflavin is both ingested in the diet and synthesized by colonic bacteria [29]. Absorption of dietary riboflavin in the upper small intestine is carrier mediated and sodium independent. The uptake mechanism is inversely regulated by extracellular thiamine levels: low serum levels upregulate uptake. Three riboflavin transporters have been identified; the most active in the gut is RFT-2 [29]. Riboflavin is exported across the basolateral membrane by a specific, electroneutral, carrier-mediated mechanism.

Vitamin C

Ascorbic acid is synthesized by most animals and acts as a cofactor in many metabolic reactions. Humans, other primates, and guinea pigs lack the active enzyme, L-gulonolactone oxidase, and cannot synthesize ascorbic acid [29]. We are thus dependent on exogenous sources.

Two transporters for vitamin C have been identified in the apical membrane: SVCT-1 and SVCT-2. These are sodium-dependent transporters that are adaptively regulated by ascorbic-acid availability [29].

Multiple choice questions

1 Sufficient intraduodenal bile acid concentration is necessary for digestion of:
   A Starch
   B Protein
   C Fat
   D Fiber
   E Glucose
2 Which of the following statements about protein digestion and absorption is *false*:
   A Protein digestion begins in the acid environment of the stomach.
   B Proteolytic enzymes are secreted by the pancreas in an active form.
   C Endopeptidases include trypsin, chymotrypsin, and elastase.
   D Exopeptidases include carboxypeptidase A and carboxypeptidase B.
   E Apical membrane-bound enzymes cleave peptides into free amino acids and di- and tripeptides that can be transported across the apical membrane.
3 Which of the following statements about carbohydrate digestion and absorption is *true*:
   A Salivary amylase produces glucose from starches.
   B Pancreatic amylase produces glucose from starches.
   C All monosaccharides are transported across the apical membrane of enterocytes by cotransport with sodium ions.

    D Intact disaccharides can be transported across the apical membrane of enterocytes.

    E Glucose, galactose, and fructose are transported out of enterocytes across the basolateral membrane by carrier-mediated facilitated diffusion via GLUT2.

4 Which of the following statements about mineral and trace element absorption is *false*:

    A Calcium and magnesium have both active and passive mechanisms of absorption.

    B Vitamin D regulates passive calcium absorption.

    C Active phosphate absorption is sodium dependent.

    D Ingested iron is taken up by enterocytes and may be stored intracellularly until hepcidin levels fall.

    E Zinc can interfere with copper absorption.

5 Fats are transported from intestinal cells to blood plasma primarily in the form of:

    A Micelles

    B Chylomicrons

    C Triglycerides

    D Fatty Acids

    E Monoglycerides

6 Triglycerides are absorbed from the lumen of the small intestine into the enterocyte as a result of:

    A Hydrolysis to free fatty acids and monoglycerides by gastric and pancreatic lipases

    B Na+ cotransport with glucose and amino acids

    C Activation of trypsinogen by enterokinase

    D An energy-dependent process utilizing ATP

References

1 Farrell, J.J. (2010) Digestion and absorption of nutrients and vitamins, in *Sleisenger & Fordtran's Gastrointestinal and Liver Disease*, 9th edn (eds M. Feldman, L. Friedman and L.J. Brandt), Saunders Elsevier, Philadelphia, pp. 1695–1734.

2 Hamosh, M. (1990) Lingual and gastric lipase. *Nutrition*, **6**, 421–428.

3 Abumrad, N.A. and Davidson, N.O. (2012) Role of the gut in lipid homeostasis. *Physiological Review*, **92**, 1061–1085.

4 Mansbach, C.M. II and Abumrad, N.A. (2012) Enterocyte fatty acid handling proteins and chylomicron formation, in *Physiology of the Gastrointestinal Tract*, 5th edn (eds L.R. Johnson, F.K. Ghishan, J.D. Kaunitz *et al.*), Academic Press Elsevier, London, pp. 1625–1641.

5 Phan, B.A.P., Dayspring, T.D. and Toth, P.P. (2012) Ezetimibe therapy: mechanism of action and clinical update. *Vascular Health and Risk Management*, **8**, 415–427.

6 De Smet, E., Mensink, R.P. and Plat, J. (2012) Effects of plant sterols and stanols on intestinal cholesterol metabolism: suggested mechanisms from past to present. *Molecular Nutrition & Food Research*, **56**, 1058–1072.

7 Ganapathy, V. (2012) Protein digestion and absorption, in *Physiology of the Gastrointestinal Tract*, 5th edn (eds L.R. Johnson, F.K. Ghishan, J.D. Kaunitz *et al.*), Academic Press Elsevier, London, pp. 1595–1623.

8 Kleinman, R.E. and Walker, W.A. (1984) Antigen processing and uptake from the intestinal tract. *Clinical Reviews in Allergy*, **2**, 25–37.

9 Wright, E.M., Sala-Rabanal, M., Loo, D.D.F. and Hirayama, B.A. (2012) Sugar absorption, in *Physiology of the Gastrointestinal Tract*, 5th edn (eds L.R. Johnson, F.K. Ghishan, J.D. Kaunitz *et al.*), Academic Press Elsevier, London, pp. 1583–1593.

10 Jones, H.F., Butler, R.N. and Brooks, D.A. (2011) Intestinal fructose transport and malabsorption in humans. *American Journal of Physiology - Gastrointestinal and Liver Physiology*, **300**, G202–G206.

11 Fine, K.D., Santa Ana, C.A., Porter, J.L. and Fordtran, J.S. (1993) Effect of D-glucose on intestinal permeability and its passive absorption in human small intestine in vivo. *Gastroenterology*, **105**, 1117–1125.

12 Fine, K.D., Santa Ana, C.A., Porter, J.L. and Fordtran, J.S. (1994) Mechanism by which glucose stimulates the passive absorption of small solutes by the human jejunum in vivo. *Gastroenterology*, **107**, 389–395.

13 Fordtran, J.S. (1975) Stimulation of active and passive sodium absorption by sugars in the human jejunum. *The Journal of Clinical Investigation*, **55**, 728–737.

14 Layden, B.T., Angueira, A.R., Brodsky, M. *et al.* (2013) Short chain fatty acids and their receptors: new metabolic targets. *Translational Research : The Journal of Laboratory and Clinical Medicine*, **161** (3), 131–140.

15 Levitt, M.D., Hirsh, P., Fetzer, C.A. *et al.* H_2 excretion after ingestion of complex carbohydrates. *Gastroenterology*, **92**, 383–389.

16 Hammer, H.F., Fine, K.D., Santa Ana, C.A. *et al.* (1990) Carbohydrate malabsorption. Its measurement and its contribution to diarrhea. *The Journal of Clinical Investigation*, **86**, 1936–1944.

17 Gill, R.K., Alrefai, W.A., Borthakur, A. and Dudeja, P.K. (2012) Intestinal anion absorption, in *Physiology of the Gastrointestinal Tract*, 5th edn (eds L.R. Johnson, F.K. Ghishan, J.D. Kaunitz *et al.*), Academic Press Elsevier, London, pp. 1819–1847.

18 Owira, P.M. and Winter, T.A. Colonic energy salvage in chronic pancreatic exocrine insufficiency. *Journal of Parenteral and Enteral Nutrition*, **32**, 63–71.

19 Kiela, P.R., Collins, J.F. and Ghishan, F.K. (2012) Molecular mechanisms of intestinal transport of calcium, phosphate, and magnesium, in *Physiology of the Gastrointestinal Tract*, 5th edn (eds L.R. Johnson, F.K. Ghishan, J.D. Kaunitz *et al.*), Academic Press Elsevier, London, pp. 1877–1919.

20 Sheikh, M.S., Schiller, L.R. and Fordtran, J.S. (1990) In vivo intestinal absorption of calcium in humans. *Mineral and Electrolyte Metabolism*, **16**, 130–146.

21 Fine, K.D., Santa Ana, C.A., Porter, J.L. and Fordtran, J.S. Intestinal absorption of magnesium from food and supplements. *Journal of Clinical Investigation*, **88**, 396–402.

22 Davis, G.R., Zerwekh, J.E., Parker, T.F. *et al.* Absorption of phosphate in the jejunum of patients with chronic renal failure before and after correction of vitamin D deficiency. *Gastroenterology*, **85**, 908–916.

23 Collins, J.E. and Anderson, G.J. (2012) Molecular mechanisms of intestinal iron transport, in *Physiology of the Gastrointestinal Tract*, 5th edn (eds L.R. Johnson, F.K. Ghishan, J.D. Kaunitz *et al.*), Academic Press Elsevier, London, pp. 1921–1947.

24 Cousins, R.J. (2012) Trace element absorption and transport, in *Physiology of the Gastrointestinal Tract*, 5th edn (eds L.R. Johnson, F.K. Ghishan, J.D Kaunitz *et al.*), Academic Press Elsevier, London, pp. 1951–1961.

25 Vavricka, S.R. and Rogler, G. Intestinal absorption and vitamin levels: is a new focus needed? *Digestive Diseases and Sciences*, **30** (Suppl 3), 73–80.

26 Cianferotti, L. and Marcocci, C. (2012) Subclinical vitamin D deficiency. *Best Practice & Research Clinical Endocrinology & Metabolism*, **26**, 523–537.

27 Pike, J.W. and Meyer, M.B. 1, 25-dihydroxyvitamin D3: synthesis, actions, and genome-scale mechanisms in the intestine and colon, in *Physiology of the Gastrointestinal Tract*, 5th edn (eds L.R. Johnson, F.K. Ghishan, J.D. Kaunitz *et al.*), Academic Press Elsevier, London, pp. 1681–1709.

28 Harrison, E.H. (2012) Digestion and intestinal absorption of dietary carotenoids and vitamin A, in *Physiology of the Gastrointestinal Tract*, 5th edn (eds L.R. Johnson, F.K. Ghishan, J.D. Kaunitz *et al.*), Academic Press Elsevier, London, pp. 1663–1680.

29 Said, H.M. and Nexo, E. (2012) Mechanisms and regulation of intestinal absorption of water-soluble vitamins: cellular and molecular aspects, in *Physiology of the Gastrointestinal Tract*, 5th edn (eds L.R. Johnson, F.K. Ghishan, J.D. Kaunitz *et al.*), Academic Press Elsevier, London, pp. 1711–1756.

Answers

1 C
2 B
3 E
4 B
5 B
6 A

CHAPTER 9

Hepatic structure and function

Michelle T. Long[1] & Lawrence S. Friedman[2,3,4,5]

[1] Boston University School of Medicine and Boston Medical Center, Boston, MA, USA
[2] Harvard Medical School, Boston, MA, USA
[3] Tufts University School of Medicine, Boston, MA, USA
[4] Massachusetts General Hospital, Boston, MA, USA
[5] Newton-Wellesley Hospital, Newton, MA, USA

Overview

A clear understanding of the structure and functional properties of the liver is necessary to fully appreciate the mechanisms behind the pathologic processes that affect the organ. This chapter reviews the gross and microscopic anatomy and major functions of the liver, in addition to providing an overview of the clinical assessment of liver function.

The liver is the largest internal organ of the human body and weighs, on average, 1500 g [1]. It is remarkably vascular; at any given time, the liver contains approximately 25% of cardiac output [2]. Before the complex nature of liver function was understood, the liver was described as a "gland," because it was known that the liver makes bile and excretes it through a centrally located system of ducts. It is preferable, however, to think of the liver as a metabolically active filter. Nutrient- and antigen-rich blood reaches the liver via the splanchnic circulation, where it is filtered through the hepatic sinusoids before entering the systemic circulation. The gross and microscopic anatomy of the liver is adapted to allow the liver to regulate the composition of blood in order to sustain the health of body tissues.

Gross anatomy

The liver sits in the right upper quadrant of the abdomen and is almost completely protected from trauma by the rib cage. It expands below the rib cage to contact the anterior abdominal wall below the right costal margin. The portion of the liver that comes in direct contact with the undersurface of the diaphragm is referred to as the *bare area*, because it is the only portion of the liver that is not covered by peritoneum. The bare area is surrounded by reflections of the parietal peritoneum that make up the superior and inferior layers of the coronary

Gastrointestinal Anatomy and Physiology: The Essentials, First Edition. Edited by John F. Reinus and Douglas Simon.
© 2014 John Wiley & Sons, Ltd. Published 2014 by John Wiley & Sons, Ltd.
www.wiley.com/go/reinus/gastro/anatomy

ligament and the right and left triangular ligaments, which attach the liver to the diaphragm. Unlike ligaments in other parts of the body, the so-called ligaments in the abdominal cavity are a double layer of peritoneum that connect the abdominal viscera together or to the abdominal wall.

Lobes

Without regard to function, the liver has traditionally been divided into four anatomic lobes: right, left, quadrate, and caudate. Anteriorly, the right lobe, which makes up five-sixths of the hepatic mass, is divided from the left lobe by the falciform ligament, which connects the liver to the anterior abdominal wall (Figure 9.1). The visceral surface of the liver is divided into the right and left lobes by the ligamentum teres, a remnant of the fetal umbilical vein along the lower border of the falciform ligament, and the ligamentum venosum, a remnant of the fetal ductus venosus that allowed maternal blood, via the umbilical vein, to bypass the fetal liver during gestation. The quadrate and caudate lobes are contiguous with the right lobe and are only visible on the visceral surface of the liver (Figure 9.2). The quadrate lobe is demarcated by the gallbladder fossa, porta hepatis, and ligamentum teres. The caudate lobe is demarcated by the inferior vena cava (IVC), porta hepatis, and ligamentum venosum. Some individuals have a downward projection of the right lobe called Riedel's lobe.

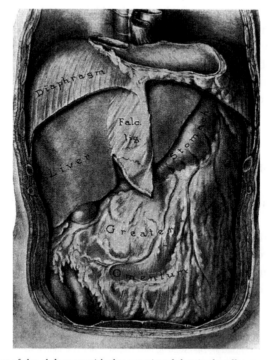

Figure 9.1 Drawing of the abdomen with the anterior abdominal wall cut away. The right and left lobes of the liver are separated by the falciform ligament. From Reference [3]. Reproduced with permission of Wolters Kluwer Health.

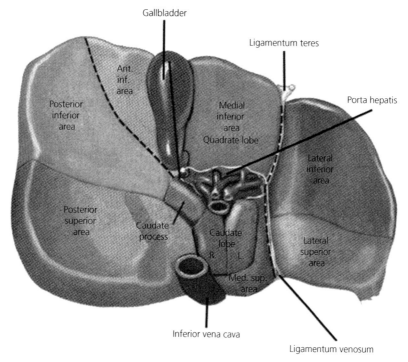

Figure 9.2 Drawing of the posterior aspect of the liver with depiction of the liver segments. The quadrate lobe is demarcated by the gallbladder, porta hepatis, and ligamentum teres. The caudate lobe is demarcated by the IVC, porta hepatis, and ligamentum venosum. The solid black line represents the "Cantlie line," which separates the functional right and left lobes. The dotted black line shows the divisions between the anterior and posterior segments of the functional right lobe and the lateral and medial segments of the functional left lobe. From Reference [4]. Reproduced with permission of Elsevier.

Segments

A more useful subdivision of the liver is made on the basis of the branching patterns of the hepatic artery, portal vein, and bile ducts, which divide the liver into right and left functional lobes. The functional right and left lobes are separated by a plane called the *Cantlie line*, which divides the liver roughly in half through the gallbladder fossa and the IVC. The right lobe is further divided into anterior and posterior segments and the left lobe into medial and lateral segments. Each of these segments is divided into superior and inferior subsegments. Several systems of subdivision have been proposed, but the most widely accepted are those of Couinaud, which follows the distribution of the portal and hepatic veins, and of Healey and Schroy, which follows the bile ducts; both systems divide the liver into eight segments [5, 6] (see Figure 9.2).

Although many connections exist between small branches of the bile ducts and afferent blood vessels in one liver segment and corresponding structures in the adjacent segments, the main bile ducts and afferent blood vessels within a liver segment do not cross the boundaries of the segment. This feature has important pathologic significance because a disturbance to a particular portal vein branch or bile duct may cause regional degeneration of a liver segment. Knowledge of the segmental anatomy of the liver is essential when planning liver surgery, but the anatomy may be difficult to discern because of a lack of intersegmental connective tissue septae. Additionally, although the branches of the hepatic artery and portal vein and the tributaries of the hepatic ducts run together to the various liver segments, the hepatic veins run independently and are intersegmental, and the major tributaries receive blood from more than one hepatic segment.

Glisson's capsule

Glisson's capsule, a thin connective tissue sheath, completely covers the liver. At the porta hepatis, the capsule thickens and extends into the parenchyma, where it merges with the connective tissue surrounding the arteries, portal veins, bile ducts, and their small branches within the portal tracts.

Vasculature

The portal vein and the hepatic artery are the two main vascular systems that supply blood to the liver. The portal vein supplies about 70% of the blood flow and 40% of the oxygen, whereas the hepatic artery supplies 30% of the blood flow and 60% of the oxygen [2]. The portal blood, which drains the mesenteric, gastric, splenic, and pancreatic veins, travels to the liver, where it branches into the right and left sides of the liver. The blood from various segments of the gastrointestinal tract in the portal system is incompletely mixed, and the relative amounts of nutrients, toxins, and other elements can vary. The hepatic artery, which arises most commonly from the celiac trunk, accompanies the portal vein at the porta hepatis, where it enters the liver and branches into the right and left sides. Small branches of the hepatic artery and portal vein feed the sinusoids and the biliary radicles. The sinusoidal blood flow is carefully regulated and collects into terminal hepatic venules before emptying into larger hepatic veins and eventually the IVC.

Microscopic anatomy

Functional units

The organization of the liver into basic functional units has been the subject of much debate since the first description of liver lobules in the seventeenth century [7]. The *classic lobule*, as described by Kiernan in 1833, is organized with a *central vein*, which is a terminal tributary of the hepatic vein, in the center and the portal tracts at three corners [8] (Figure 9.3). This organization differs from the lobular architecture of glands, which is centered around ducts instead of blood vessels.

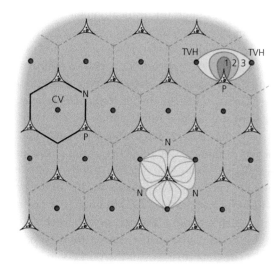

Figure 9.3 Schematic drawing of liver architecture. At the left is the classic hepatic lobule, with the central vein as its center and portal tracts at three corners. In the middle toward the bottom is the portal lobule, with the portal tract at its center and central veins and nodal points at its periphery. At the right is the liver acinus, the center of which is the terminal afferent vessel (in the portal tract) and the periphery of which is drained by the terminal hepatic venule, or central vein. Zones 1, 2, and 3 extending from the portal tract to the terminal hepatic venule are shown. CV, central vein; N, nodal point; P, portal tract; TVH, terminal hepatic venule. From Reference [9]. Reproduced with permission of Elsevier.

In 1906, Mall described the *portal lobule* with the portal tract in the center and the central veins at the periphery. This model allows the draining duct and blood supply to be central, as they are in true glands [10] (see Figure 9.3). Although this organization is more consistent with the organization of other tissues, it has little functional significance.

In 1954, Rappaport offered an alternative unit to the portal lobule by defining the *liver acinus*, which was the first attempt to describe the structure of the liver unit as it relates to function [11]. The liver acinus is a globular array of hepatocytes around a small portal tract containing a bile ductule, terminal portal vein, and hepatic arteriole, the latter two of which supply this group of hepatocytes with blood. At the periphery of the liver acinus lie the central veins (from the classic lobule), which drain the area (see Figure 9.3). In this model, three hepatic parenchymal zones are described that divide groups of hepatocytes according to their relative distance from the oxygen-rich portal tract. The periportal zone (zone 1) receives blood with the highest oxygen and nutrient content, followed by the intermediate zone (zone 2), and lastly the perivenular zone (zone 3), which is closest to the terminal hepatic (central) veins and receives the most oxygen-poor blood. The concept of the liver acinus, with the incorporation of both a structural and functional organization, has been of great value because it facilitates the description of important histopathologic features, such as portal–central bridging, hepatic necrosis, and fibrosis.

The major criticism of the liver acinus model is that it is not based on actual vascular reconstruction. In 1982, Matsumoto and Kawakami presented another view of the liver functional unit based on its angioarchitecture that more closely resembles the classic lobule [12]. In this *primary lobule* model, the portal and hepatic venous systems are divided into a conduction portion, which delivers and drains blood from the parenchyma, and a parenchymal portion, which consists of three levels of minute side branches of the portal and hepatic veins. Branches of the portal and hepatic veins arise in orderly rows from each terminal branch of the conduction portion. Additional branches of the portal and hepatic veins arise from these primary branches, although the portal vein branches are more numerous so that about six portal vein branches supply an area of parenchyma with one hepatic vein at the center (mimicking the classic lobule with a central vein). The final divisions of the portal venous system are called septal branches. The primary lobule is defined as a conical cluster of hepatocytes that receives blood through the septal branches and is drained by multiple venules that ultimately feed into a central vein. In this model, the oxygen-rich blood from the portal tract forms a sickle-shaped front of blood flow with the convex aspect abutting a portal tract and the concave aspect facing the central vein (Figure 9.4).

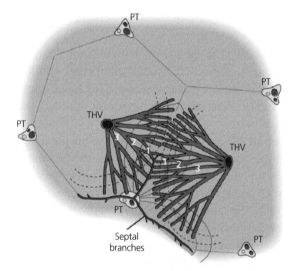

Figure 9.4 Drawing that compares liver blood flow in the three zones of the acinus model with Matsumoto's concept of liver architecture. According to the model by Matsumoto, sinusoids that abut portal tracts and terminal afferent vessels (septal branches) form a hemodynamically equipotential sickle-shaped perfusion front (*dotted lines*). This model conforms to the concept of the classic lobule rather than to the acinus. Zones 1, 2, and 3 of the hepatic acinus are labeled. PT, portal tract; THV, terminal hepatic venule. From Reference [9]. Reproduced with permission of Elsevier.

Portal tracts

The portal tract (or triad) contains small branches of the hepatic artery and portal vein, an interlobular bile duct, nerve fibers, and fine lymphatics that are all surrounded by a perivascular fibrous connective tissue capsule that extends from Glisson's capsule and provides a framework for the hepatic parenchyma. The hepatic parenchyma immediately surrounding the portal space, the *periportal area*, is not in direct communication with the portal structures. The *limiting plate*, a continuous barrier of hepatocytes surrounding the portal area, has small openings for the terminal hepatic arterioles and portal venules that supply mixed arterial and portal blood to the sinusoids. The hepatic arterioles give off branches to form a dense capillary network called the *periductal plexus,* which surrounds the bile ductules and drains into the sinusoids. The existence of the periductal plexus suggests the possibility of an exchange mechanism between arterial blood and bile ductules.

Sinusoids

The hepatic sinusoids are a complex network of vascular spaces that are sandwiched between liver cell (hepatocyte) plates (Figure 9.5). As described earlier, blood from the terminal branches of the portal vasculature that exits the portal

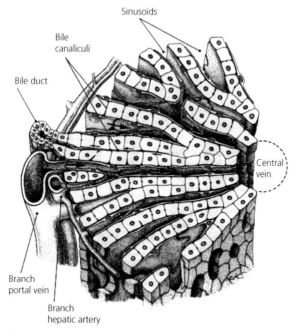

Figure 9.5 Radial distribution of the liver cell (hepatocyte) plates and sinusoids around the terminal hepatic venule, or central vein. A bile duct, branches of the portal vein hepatic artery, and bile canaliculi are shown. From Reference [13]. Reproduced with permission of Hodder Education.

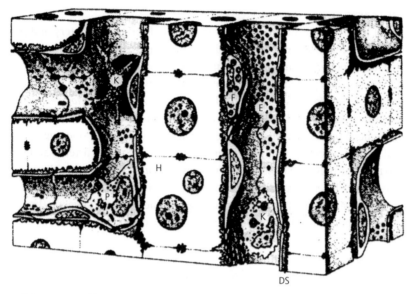

Figure 9.6 Drawing of liver cell plates and adjoining sinusoids. DS, space of Disse;
E, endothelial cell; F, stellate (fat-storing, Ito) cell; H, hepatocyte; K, Kupffer cell;
P, pit cell. From Reference [14]. Reproduced with permission of S. Karger AG, Basel.

area through the limiting plate perfuses the hepatic sinusoids, which transfer
mixed arterial and portal blood to the central veins.

Hepatic sinusoids are composed of four cell types: endothelial, Kupffer,
stellate, and pit cells (Figure 9.6). *Endothelial cells*, which contain the sinusoids,
are the primary barrier between blood and hepatocytes. These endothelial cells
are unique in that they contain numerous fenestrations, lack a basement membrane, and can transfer molecules via endocytosis [15]. The fenestrations are
clustered in small patches called *sieve plates* and lack diaphragms. Endothelial
cells filter fluids, solutes, and particles between blood and the *space of Disse*, which
overlies the liver cell plate and contains an ultrafiltrate of blood. The porosity of
the endothelial cell is greatest in the perivenular area because endothelial cell
fenestrae are more numerous and larger near the central veins [16]. *Kupffer cells*
are macrophages within the sinusoidal lumen that are attached to endothelial
cells. These phagocytic cells clear the blood of senescent red blood cells and
toxic substances. Kupffer cells are larger and more phagocytically active in the
periportal areas, where they serve as a first line of defense against pathogens
[15]. They can proliferate locally and are also the major producers of cytokines
that serve as mediators of inflammation. *Pit cells* are a special hepatic population
of large granular lymphocytes anchored to the sinusoidal endothelium by pseu-
dopodia. *Stellate cells* (also known as fat-storing cells, lipocytes, or Ito cells) are
mesenchymal cells located in the space of Disse and surround the sinusoidal

lumens; they are sites of fat metabolism. Chronic inflammation activates stellate cells, which transform into myofibroblasts.

Hepatocytes and liver cell plates

Hepatocytes are polyhedral cells with rounded nuclei of various sizes; up to 25% of hepatocytes are binucleated. The surface area of hepatocytes is increased by abundant microvilli. The majority of the hepatic parenchyma is composed of an interconnecting network of hepatocytes arranged in *liver cell plates*, which are separated by sinusoids (see Figure 9.5). These plates are usually one and occasionally two cells thick, so that each hepatocyte is in direct contact with another hepatocyte, an intervening bile canaliculus, and the space of Disse. The liver cell plates are supported by a reticulin network that forms the skeleton of the hepatic parenchyma and is continuous with the perivascular fibrous capsule surrounding the vessels in the portal area.

Hepatocytes display *structural heterogeneity*, reflecting their functional diversity. Therefore, periportal hepatocytes differ from perivenular hepatocytes in the ratio of surface area to the volume of adjacent sinusoids, as well as in certain subcellular features such as the numbers of Golgi complexes and lysosomes and the quantity of smooth endoplasmic reticulum. This diversity is believed to be a response to the microenvironment of the hepatocyte, rather than an expression of fundamental developmental differences.

Space of Disse and lymph

Hepatocytes are separated from the sinusoids by the *space of Disse* (see Figure 9.6). Plasma passes freely from the sinusoidal lumen through the fenestrations in the endothelial cells and into the space of Disse, where it comes into direct contact with the hepatocyte surface. Plasma circulates through the space of Disse and flows toward the central vein; however, some plasma is taken up by the lymphatic spaces in the periportal area and may reenter sinusoidal blood. There are no lymphatics within the liver lobule. The liver produces 25–50% of the lymph passing through the thoracic duct. Hepatic lymph contains more protein than does lymph from other parts of the body.

Bile canaliculi and ducts

A *bile canaliculus* is located between each adjacent pair of hepatocytes (see Figure 9.5). The canaliculi form a network of interconnected channels throughout the hepatic parenchyma. The canalicular wall is formed by a specialized portion of the liver cell membrane covered with microvilli, and the lumen is completely isolated from the intercellular space, including the space of Disse, by junctional complexes.

Bile flows from the canaliculi through the *canals of Hering*, which are openings in the limiting plate, into the smallest biliary radicles, known as the portal *bile ductules*, or *cholangioles*. The bile ductules and the larger bile ducts are lined by *cholangiocytes*. Bile ductules join together to form interlobular and then septal bile ducts; several successive orders of septal bile ducts ultimately merge into the right and left hepatic ducts, which, in turn, join to form the common hepatic duct near the liver hilum. Bile ductules, interlobular bile ducts, and first- and second-generation septal bile ducts comprise the *small-duct biliary system*. Larger septal bile ducts, segmental bile ducts, the hepatic ducts, and the bile duct (common bile duct) comprise the *large-duct biliary system*.

Hepatic veins

As described earlier, the terminal branch of the hepatic vein is referred to as the central vein because of its location in the center of the classic lobule. Sinusoidal blood flows into central veins. The central veins do not have a fibrous capsule like the portal vessels, and therefore, they are not isolated from the hepatic parenchyma. Small central veins coalesce into larger intersegmental branches of the right, left, and middle hepatic veins. The right, middle, and left hepatic veins deliver deoxygenated blood to the IVC. The right hepatic vein typically enters the IVC separately, but the middle hepatic and left hepatic veins may share a common trunk in up to 85% of patients [17]. Additionally, small accessory hepatic veins, particularly in the right lobe, are common. Knowledge of anatomic variations in venous drainage is particularly important in planning liver surgery.

Innervation

The liver is innervated by preganglionic parasympathetic fibers derived from the anterior and posterior vagi and postganglionic sympathetic fibers from the celiac ganglia [18]. These nerve fibers reach the liver via two intercommunicating plexi around the hepatic artery and portal vein. The importance of the hepatic nervous system is unclear, because denervated orthotopic liver allografts function well despite little reinnervation [19].

Function

Sinusoids

The hepatic sinusoid is not merely a passive conduit; sinusoidal cells perform a number of important physiologic functions. They are active in both receptor- and nonreceptor-mediated endocytosis, secrete bioactive lipids and cytokines, have cytotoxic activity, produce collagen, and are the gatekeepers for the intra-hepatic filtration of portal blood.

The hepatic *sinusoidal endothelium* is highly permeable to plasma solutes. The endothelial fenestrae measure 150–200 nm in diameter and occupy 6–8% of the endothelial surface [20]. Because of the fenestrations in the sinusoidal endothelial cells and the absence of covering diaphragms or a basement membrane, there is no barrier to filtration of macromolecules up to 250 000 daltons in weight or of particles up to 0.2 μm in diameter. Chylomicron remnants and very-low-density lipoprotein particles can traverse the sinusoidal endothelium freely and gain entry into the space of Disse. Direct contact between plasma solutes and the absorptive surfaces of hepatocytes facilitates exchange of materials between blood and the liver cell. The movement of fluids, solutes, and particles is bidirectional, allowing an intensive interaction between the sinusoidal blood and the microvillus surface of the parenchymal cells [16]. Additionally, differences in the diameter and frequency of fenestrae exist between the periportal and the centrilobular zones: the sinusoid becomes more porous as it reaches the centrilobular area [16]. The fenestrae are dynamic structures the diameter and number of which vary in response to a variety of hormones, drugs, toxins, and diseases and even to changes in the underlying extracellular matrix. Various hepatotoxins, including ethanol, induce defenestration of the endothelial membrane, which occurs early in the pathogenesis of cirrhosis [21].

Movement of fluid and solutes out of the sinusoidal lumen is dependent primarily on the pressure gradient between the intravascular space and the space of Disse. The elevation of intrasinusoidal pressure in many forms of portal hypertension tends to force more fluid and solute out of the hepatic sinusoid, and when the volume of material is too great to be returned to the systemic circulation by the lymphatics, the fluid weeps off the surface of the liver and may accumulate in the peritoneal cavity as ascites.

Sinusoidal endothelial cells also secrete bioactive compounds, including prostaglandin E2, prostacyclin, cytokines, and nitric oxide (NO), and are involved in the secretion of the extracellular matrix [22]. In addition, they are actively engaged in endocytosis and are therefore a part of the reticuloendothelial system along with Kupffer and pit cells.

Kupffer cells, the largest population of tissue macrophages in the mononuclear phagocyte system, are strategically located within hepatic sinusoids to survey the filtered portal blood for the presence of a variety of foreign substances. Kupffer cells engage in endocytosis of microbial organisms, enzymes, tumor cells, antigens, and immune complexes. They are the principal site for clearance of endotoxin from portal blood and display the highest capacity of any tissue macrophage for detoxifying endotoxin. Kupffer cells act as antigen-processing cells, sequestering some antigens, for example, dietary proteins, to prevent initiation of an immune response, and acting as antigen-presenting cells to induce an immune response to other antigens. When activated by the proper stimuli, Kupffer cells release bioactive lipids (prostaglandins and leukotrienes) and peptides (interleukins, interferon, and tumor necrosis factor), which play a central role in immune and inflammatory reactions. They also participate in these reactions by killing tumor cells and intracellular protozoan parasites. Finally, Kupffer cells are responsible for the clearance of senescent erythrocytes and the degradation of hemoglobin. There is evidence to suggest *functional heterogeneity* of Kupffer cells: periportal Kupffer cells are more numerous and larger, have more lysosomes, and display more phagocytic activity, but less tumor cytotoxic potential, than do Kupffer cells in acinar zones 2 and 3.

Pit cells are another group of immune effector cells that reside in hepatic sinusoids. Pit cells are non-B and non-T cells of natural killer cell lineage responsible for killing tumor cells and cells infected with virus particles.

Stellate cells, also located in the sinusoids, have four main functions in the liver. First, they produce extracellular matrix proteins and, when stimulated by inflammatory mediators, transform into myofibroblasts, which synthesize a diverse array of connective tissue components including collagen types I, III, and IV, fibronectin, laminin, dermatan sulfate, chondroitin sulfate, and tenascin [23]. Stellate cells are considered the major contributor to matrix homeostasis within the liver parenchyma. Second, stellate cells play a role in hepatic regeneration, both in the normal liver and in response to injury. They secrete a variety of growth factors, including hepatocyte growth factor, which stimulates parenchymal cell proliferation, and transforming growth factor-β, which inhibits parenchymal cell proliferation and stimulates connective tissue synthesis. Third, stellate cells are thought to play a role in the control of vascular tone. Positioned around the sinusoidal membrane, stellate cells can regulate sinusoidal blood flow in response to stimulation by endothelins and nitric oxide [23]. The final major function of stellate cells is in the storage of vitamin A. Dietary retinyl esters are taken up by hepatocytes, which transfer the majority of the endocytosed retinol to the stellate cells. As with the other sinusoidal cells, evidence of functional heterogeneity of stellate cells exists, and the greatest number is found in the periportal area.

Hepatocytes

Hepatocytes comprise 80% of the cytoplasmic mass of the liver and are the site of major liver functions, including nutrient metabolism, synthesis and degradation of plasma proteins, detoxification of xenobiotic compounds, and bile formation. Variations exist in the ability of hepatocytes in different hepatic zones to perform some of these functions (functional heterogeneity).

Hepatocytes play a pivotal role in nutrient metabolism and, therefore, in energy and nitrogen balance, the determining factors in the functional and structural integrity of the organism. They regulate energy and nitrogen balance by uptake and release of glucose and amino acids, glycogen synthesis and storage, processing of lipids, and production of ketone bodies and urea. Hepatocytes differ in the amounts and activities of the rate-limiting enzymes involved in carbohydrate and oxidative metabolism and, therefore, in their metabolic capacities. Periportal hepatocytes are mainly responsible for oxidative catabolism of fatty and amino acids and also for glucose release and glycogen formation through gluconeogenesis. Perivenous hepatocytes use glucose primarily for the synthesis of glycogen and for glycolysis coupled to liponeogenesis. Similar differences exist between periportal and perivenous hepatocytes with respect to their capacities for ammonia and amino acid metabolism. Hepatocytes in the periportal zone have a high capacity for uptake and catabolism of most amino acids and also for urea synthesis. Perivenous cells are mainly active in glutamine synthesis and remove ammonia that has escaped metabolism to urea in the periportal area from sinusoidal blood. This form of functional heterogeneity allows the liver to play an important role in acid–base homeostasis.

Another major hepatocyte function is the synthesis and degradation of plasma proteins, including those that maintain plasma oncotic pressure (albumin), serve as carrier molecules (albumin, transferrin, ceruloplasmin, haptoglobin, lipoproteins), inhibit proteases (albumin, α_1-antitrypsin, α_2-macroglobulin), act as intercellular messengers (hormones, prohormones), and participate in hemostasis (coagulation factors, regulatory proteins, fibrinolytic proteins). The coagulopathy that may complicate acute or chronic liver disease is caused not only by impaired synthesis of clotting factors (II, V, VII, IX, X, XIII) but also by decreased synthesis of contact activation factors (XI, XII, prekallikrein, high-molecular-weight kininogen), fibrinolytic factors (plasminogen), and regulatory proteins (α_2-antiplasmin, α_2-macroglobulin, antithrombin) and by decreased hepatic clearance and degradation of activated factors. All hepatocytes are engaged in protein metabolism; whether or not different areas of the liver display functional heterogeneity in the synthesis and degradation of plasma proteins is unclear.

Hepatocytes are the cells responsible for the detoxification of xenobiotic compounds, most notably drugs. Hepatocytes contain the cytochrome P450 enzymes, a heterogeneous group of proteins that catalyze the oxidation and reduction reactions of the first step in the biotransformation of drugs (phase 1 metabolism). The multiple forms of the cytochrome P450 enzymes are the products of a gene superfamily. Three gene families (I, II, III) within the superfamily code for the enzymes that are important in human drug metabolism. Cytochrome P450 II is the largest family of human cytochrome enzymes; transcription and translation of the subfamily, P450 IIE, is induced by ingestion of ethanol or isoniazid. The P450 III family codes for the enzymes responsible for phase 1 metabolism of anticonvulsant drugs.

The metabolites of the cytochrome P450 enzymes may retain some drug activity or be toxic and, therefore, must be eliminated from the body. After completion of phase 1 metabolism, drug metabolites are conjugated by hepatocytes to glucuronic acid, sulfate, or glutathione (phase 2 metabolism), thereby making them water soluble so that they can be excreted in the bile or urine.

Bile formation and excretion is one of the most important functions of the hepatocyte. This topic is covered at length in Chapter 11.

Assessment of liver function

There is no single test or group of tests that serves to accurately evaluate the many functions of the liver. The term "liver function tests" is a misnomer because serum levels of the most commonly measured substances, the aminotransferases and alkaline phosphatase, are not quantitatively related to a function of the liver. Therefore, the term liver biochemical tests may be more appropriate [24]. Levels of serum bilirubin and serum albumin and the prothrombin time are reflections of liver function but also are influenced by many factors extrinsic to the liver. Abnormal liver biochemical test results are often the first indication of clinical or subclinical liver disease. Analysis of the pattern of abnormalities frequently suggests a specific category of liver injury, even a specific diagnosis; however, normal or minimally abnormal liver biochemical test levels do not exclude serious liver disease, such as advanced cirrhosis. Laboratory test results, particularly those used to calculate the Model for End-Stage Liver Disease score, may provide information about the severity of liver damage and thus prognosis; sequential testing may allow assessment of the effectiveness of therapy.

Aminotransferases

The serum aminotransferases are intracellular enzymes released from damaged hepatocytes and, as such, are useful markers of hepatic injury. Aspartate aminotransferase (AST) (formerly serum glutamic oxaloacetic transaminase (SGOT)) is found in both the cytosol and mitochondria of hepatocytes as well as in the skeletal muscle, heart, kidney, brain, and pancreas. AST has a serum half-life of about 18 h. Alanine aminotransferase (ALT) (formerly serum glutamic pyruvate transaminase (SGPT)) is found only in the cytosol and has the highest concentration in the liver, thereby making it more sensitive and specific than AST as a marker of liver inflammation or necrosis. ALT has a serum half-life of approximately 48 h. A serum aminotransferase elevation is often the first biochemical abnormality detected in patients with viral, autoimmune, or drug hepatitis, but the degree of elevation does not correlate well with the extent of hepatic injury (Table 9.1) [24].

The ratio of AST to ALT in serum can be helpful in suggesting the underlying cause of liver damage. For example, in alcoholic hepatitis, the serum AST level is usually no more than two to five times the upper limit of normal, and the ALT level is usually near normal and may be normal. The relatively low serum ALT level may be the result of a deficiency of pyridoxal-5-phosphate, a necessary cofactor for hepatic synthesis of ALT. In addition, alcohol-induced liver injury leads to increased release of mitochondrial AST. In this condition, the AST:ALT ratio is typically greater than two. By contrast, the serum ALT level is greater than the AST level in nonalcoholic fatty liver, nonalcoholic steatohepatitis, and

Table 9.1 Causes of serum aminotransferase elevations[a].

Mild elevations (≤5× normal)	Severe elevations (≥15× normal)
Hepatic: ALT predominant	Acute viral hepatitis (A–E, herpes virus)
Chronic hepatitis B, C, and D	Ischemic hepatitis
Acute viral hepatitis (A–E, EBV, CMV)	Autoimmune hepatitis
Steatosis/steatohepatitis	Wilson's disease
Hemochromatosis	Acute bile duct obstruction
Medications/toxins	Acute Budd–Chiari syndrome
Autoimmune hepatitis	Hepatic artery ligation
Alpha-1 antitrypsin deficiency	
Wilson's disease	
Celiac disease	
Glycogenic hepatopathy	
Hepatic: AST predominant	
Alcohol-related liver injury (AST:ALT > 2:1)	
Cirrhosis	
Nonhepatic	
Hemolysis	
Macro-AST	
Myopathy	
Strenuous exercise	
Thyroid disease	

[a]Virtually any liver disease can cause moderate aminotransferase elevations (5–15× normal).
ALT, alanine aminotransferase; AST, aspartate aminotransferase; CMV, cytomegalovirus; EBV, Epstein–Barr virus.

viral hepatitis, although the AST:ALT ratio often rises to greater than one as cirrhosis develops, possibly because of reduced clearance of AST [25]. The degree of aminotransferase elevation can be helpful in determining the underlying etiology of hepatic injury. Aminotransferase levels may be greater than 1000 U/l in acute or chronic viral hepatitis, drug-induced liver injury, autoimmune hepatitis, and acute Budd–Chiari syndrome. In acetaminophen-induced fulmi-nant hepatic failure and ischemic hepatopathy, higher values (>5000 U/l) may be found (Table 9.1), and the ratio of AST to ALT tends to resemble that seen in patients with alcoholic hepatitis.

Alkaline phosphatase

Alkaline phosphatase is an enzyme bound to the hepatic canalicular membrane and functions to detoxify lipopolysaccharide, protect the intestinal barrier, and hydrolyze phosphate esters to generate inorganic phosphate for uptake by various tissues. Alkaline phosphatase is a sensitive test for detecting both intra- and extrahepatic biliary tract obstruction. Increases in the serum alkaline phosphatase level appear to result from increased hepatic synthesis of the enzyme, which may be promoted by increases in bile acid concentrations in the liver. Alkaline phosphatase is also found in the bone, intestine, kidney, and placenta, and striking elevations can be seen with Paget's disease of the bone, osteoblastic bone metastases, and small bowel obstruction. Moderate elevations are seen in normal pregnancy and with rapid bone growth in children. An hepatic origin of an elevated serum alkaline phosphatase level is suggested by simultaneous elevation of the serum level of alkaline phosphatase and either the serum 5'-nucleotidase, which is relatively specific to the liver, or the gamma glutamyl transpeptidase, which is more sensitive than the 5'-nucleotidase. An isolated elevation of the serum alkaline phosphatase of hepatic origin may indicate an infiltrative liver disease caused by a tumor, abscess, granulomatous disease, or amyloidosis. High serum levels of alkaline phosphatase are associated with biliary obstruction, sclerosing cholangitis, immunoglobulin (Ig) G_4-associated cholangitis, primary biliary cirrhosis, and overlap syndromes [26]. Patients with chronic hepatitis or cirrhosis often have mild elevations of the serum alkaline phosphatase. Alkaline phosphatase has a relatively long half-life of about seven days, and levels may remain elevated up to one week after relief of biliary obstruction and the return of the serum bilirubin level to normal.

Bilirubin

Elevations in the serum bilirubin level are manifested clinically by jaundice when the level exceeds 3 mg/dl. Bilirubin is formed primarily as a degradation product of hemoglobin. Following red blood cell breakdown in the reticuloendothelial system, heme is cleaved by the enzyme heme oxygenase to form iron, carbon monoxide, and biliverdin. Biliverdin is converted to bilirubin, which is released into the blood and transported to the liver tightly bound to albumin. This free, or unconjugated, bilirubin is lipid soluble and is not filtered by the glomerulus. Unconjugated bilirubin is taken up by the liver, presumably by organic anion transport proteins on the basolateral membranes of hepatocytes, and attaches to intracellular storage proteins (ligandins). The bilirubin is then conjugated to a diglucuronide and, to a lesser extent, a monoglucuronide by the enzyme uridine diphosphate-glucuronyl transferase. Water-soluble, conjugated bilirubin is excreted into bile against a steep concentration gradient by the canalicular multispecific organic anion transporter, also referred to as the multidrug resistance-associated protein 2. Defects in one of a number of hepatocanalicular transporters (primarily ATP-binding

Table 9.2 Causes of conjugated hyperbilirubinemia.

Intrahepatic cholestasis
Cirrhosis
Drugs (e.g., oral contraceptives in heterozygotes for multidrug resistance 3 transporter deficiency)
Hepatitis
Intrahepatic cholestasis of pregnancy
Primary biliary cirrhosis
Sepsis
Total parenteral nutrition
Extrahepatic biliary obstruction
Biliary atresia
Choledocholithiasis
Neoplasm
Parasitic infection
Sclerosing cholangitis
Stricture

cassette [ABC] transporters) result in a variety of genetic and familial chole-static syndromes [27]. Bilirubin is hydrolyzed by β-glucuronidases to form unconjugated bilirubin in the distal ileum and colon. Unconjugated bilirubin is then reduced by intestinal bacteria to colorless urobilinogens and their colored derivatives, urobilins, which are excreted in feces (Chapter 11).

Hyperbilirubinemia may be classified based on whether or not the excess bilirubin is conjugated to glucuronic acid. Unconjugated hyperbilirubinemia can result from overproduction, such that the quantity of bilirubin exceeds the hepatic capacity for uptake and conjugation, as in hemolysis, ineffective erythropoiesis, and the resorption of a hematoma. Alternatively, serum uncon-jugated bilirubin levels may be elevated in the setting of defective conjugation of bilirubin to glucuronide in patients with Gilbert syndrome. Conjugated hyperbilirubinemia can result from rare genetic disorders of hepatocanalicular transport, as in Dubin–Johnson syndrome, Rotor syndrome, benign recurrent intrahepatic cholestasis, and progressive familial intrahepatic cholestasis (PFIC) [27]. More commonly, elevations of serum conjugated bilirubin levels can be seen in disorders associated with hepatocellular injury, intrahepatic cholestasis, or extrahepatic biliary obstruction (Table 9.2).

Serum proteins

Most proteins that circulate in the plasma are synthesized by hepatocytes, and the levels of proteins in the blood reflect the synthetic capability of the liver. Albumin accounts for 10% of hepatic protein synthesis and 75% of protein in serum. Hypoalbuminemia may result from expanded plasma volume, as in pregnancy, which decreases the concentration of albumin, or from decreased hepatic synthesis; it is a common feature of chronic liver disease [28].

Serum globulins are often increased in chronic liver disease, and their pattern of elevation may suggest the etiology of the underlying disorder. For example, an elevated IgG level in serum is associated with autoimmune hepatitis, whereas elevations in IgM and IgA levels are associated with primary biliary cirrhosis and alcoholic liver disease, respectively.

The majority of the coagulation factors, with the exception of factor VIII, are synthesized in the liver, and deficiencies of these factors in patients with liver disease lead to prolongation of the prothrombin time. The prothrombin time is useful in assessing the severity and prognosis of liver disease but correlates poorly with bleeding risk because of counterbalancing disturbances in anticoagulant activity [29]. Advanced chronic liver disease, in fact, is now considered to be a prothrombotic state [29].

Acknowledgment

The authors thank John F. Reinus, MD, for his contribution of a previous version of this chapter.

Multiple choice questions

1 In which of the following descriptions of the basic functional unit of the liver is the terminal hepatic venule (the central vein) located in the center?
   A Classic lobule
   B Portal lobule
   C Liver acinus
   D Primary lobule
   E A and C
   F A and D

2 Functions of the hepatic stellate cell include all of the following *except*:
   A Production of extracellular matrix proteins
   B Secretion of growth factors
   C Synthesis of coagulation factors
   D Control of vascular tone
   E Storage of vitamin A

3 Which of the following conditions typically causes elevations in serum aminotransferase levels >1000 U/l?
   A Alcoholic liver disease
   B Celiac disease
   C Chronic hepatitis C
   D Autoimmune hepatitis
   E Nonalcoholic fatty liver disease

4 Concerning sinusoidal function, which statement is correct?

   A Kupffer cells are tissue macrophages which process antigens, release a range of bioactive amines, and clear senescent red blood cells.

   B Pit cells store and metabolize fat and when stimulated change into myofibroblasts.

   C The sinusoidal endothelium has tight junctions between them and limits access to the space of Disse.

   D Movement of fluid and solutes into the space of Disse and therefore to the hepatocytes is regulated by active exchange pumps.

5 Concerning hepatocyte function, which statement is correct?

   A Hepatocytes play a role in nutrient metabolism, nitrogen, and energy balance.

   B Hepatocytes show functional heterogeneity based on their location in the hepatic zone.

   C Most clotting factors are made in the liver.

   D All are true.

References

1 Skandalakis, J.E., Skandalakis, L.J., Skandalakis, P.N. and Mirilas, P. (2004) Hepatic surgical anatomy. *The Surgical Clinics of North America*, **84**, 413–435.

2 Burt, A.D. and Day, C.P. (2003) Pathophysiology of the liver, in *Pathology of the Liver*, 4th edn (ed. R. MacSween), Churchill Livingstone, New York, pp. 67–105.

3 Grant, J.C.B. (1972) *An Atlas of Anatomy*, 6th edn, Williams and Wilkins, Baltimore, p. 125.

4 Netter, F.H. (1997) *Atlas of Human Anatomy*, 3rd edn, Novartis, New Jersey.

5 Couinaud, C. (1957) *Le Foie. Etudes Anatomiques et Chirurgicales*, Masson & Cie, Paris.

6 Healey, J.J. and Schroy, P. (1953) Anatomy of the biliary ducts within the human liver: analysis of the prevailing pattern of branching and the major variations of the biliary ducts. *Archives of Surgery*, **66**, 599–616.

7 Bloch, E.H. (1970) The termination of hepatic arterioles and the functional unit of the liver as determined by microscopy of the living organ. *Annals of the New York Academy of Sciences*, **170**, 78–87.

8 Kiernan, F. (1833) The anatomy and physiology of the liver. *Philosophical Transactions of the Royal Society of London*, **123**, 711–770.

9 Misdraji, J. (2010) Anatomy, histology, embryology, and developmental anomalies of the liver, in *Sleisenger and Fordtran's Gastrointestinal and Liver Disease: Pathophysiology/Diagnosis/ Management*, 9th edn (eds M. Feldman, L.S. Friedman and L.J. Brandt), Saunders Elsevier, Philadelphia, pp. 1201–1206.

10 Mall, F.P. (1906) A study of the functional unit of the liver. *American Journal of Anatomy*, **5**, 227–308.

11 Rappaport, A.M., Borowy, Z.J., Lougheed, W.M. and Lotto, W.N. (1954) Subdivision of hexagonal liver lobules into a structural and functional unit. Role in hepatic physiology and pathology. *The Anatomical Record*, **119**, 11–34.

12 Matsumoto, T. and Kawakami, M. (1982) The unit-concept of hepatic parenchyma – a re-examination based on angioarchitectural studies. *Acta Pathologica Japonica*, **32** (Suppl 2), 285–314.

13 Fawcett, D.W. (1997) *Bloom and Fawcett: A Textbook of Histology*, 12th edn, Hodder Arnold, London.

14 Sasse, D., Spornitz, U.M. and Maly, I.P. (1992) Liver architecture. *Enzyme*, **46**, 8–32.

15 Malarkey DE, Johnson, K., Ryan, L. *et al.* (2004) New insights into functional aspects of liver morphology. *Toxicologic Pathology*, **33**, 27–34.

16 Braet, F. and Wisse, E. (2002) Structural and functional aspects of liver sinusoidal endothelial cell fenestrae: a review. *Comparative Hepatology*, **1**, 1.

17 Cheng, Y.F., Huang, T.L., Chen, C.L. *et al.* (1997) Variations of the middle and inferior right hepatic vein: application in hepatectomy. *Journal of Clinical Ultrasound*, **25**, 175–182.

18 Roskam T., Desmet, V.J., Verstype, C.. (2007) Development, structure and function of the liver, in *Pathology of the Liver*, 5th edn (ed. R. MacSween), Churchill Livingstone, New York, pp. 2–61.

19 Saxena R, Theise, N.D. and Crawford, J.M. (1999) Microanatomy of the human liver-exploring the hidden interfaces. *Hepatology*, **30**, 1339–1346.

20 Wisse, E., De Zanger, R.B., Charels, K. *et al.* (1985) The liver sieve: considerations concerning the structure and function of endothelial fenestrae, the sinusoidal wall and the space of Disse. *Hepatology*, **5**, 683–689.

21 Dobbs, B.R., Rogers, G.W.T., Xing, H.Y. and Fraser, R. (1994) Endotoxin-induced defenestration of the hepatic sinusoidal endothelium: a factor in the pathogenesis of cirrhosis? *Liver*, **14**, 230–233.

22 Shah, V., Garcia-Gardena, G., Sessa, W.C. and Groszmann, R.J. (1998) The hepatic circulation in health and disease: a report of a single-topic symposium. *Hepatology*, **27**, 279–288.

23 Burt, A.D. (1999) Pathobiology of the hepatic stellate cells. *Journal of Gastroenterology*, **34**, 299–304.

24 Friedman, L.S., Martin, P. and Muñoz, S.J. (2003) Liver function tests and the objective evaluation of the patient with liver disease, in *Hepatology: A Textbook of Liver Disease*, 4th edn (eds D. Zakim and T.D. Boyer), Saunders, Philadelphia, pp. 661–708.

25 Sorbi, D., Boynton, J. and Lindor, K.D. (1999) The ratio of aspartate aminotransferase to alanine aminotransferase: potential value in differentiating nonalcoholic steatohepatitis from alcoholic liver disease. *The American journal of Gastroenterology*, **94**, 1018–1022.

26 Heathcote, E.J. (2007) Diagnosis and management of cholestatic liver disease. *Clinical Gastroenterology and Hepatology*, **5**, 776–782.

27 Oude Elferink, R.P.J., Paulusma, C.C. and Groen, A.K. (2006) Hepatocanalicular transport defects: pathophysiologic mechanisms of rare diseases. *Gastroenterology*, **130**, 908–925.

28 Quinlan, G.J., Martin, G.S. and Evans, T.W. (2005) Albumin: biochemical properties and therapeutic potential. *Hepatology*, **41**, 1211–1219.

29 Tripodi, A. and Mannucci, P.M. (2011) The coagulopathy of chronic liver disease. *The New England Journal of Medicine*, **365**, 147–156.

Answers

1 F
2 C
3 D
4 A
5 D

CHAPTER 10

The splanchnic circulation

Peter R. Kvietys[1] & D. Neil Granger[2]

[1] *College of Medicine, Alfaisal University, Riyadh, Saudi Arabia*
[2] *Department of Molecular & Cellular Physiology, LSU Health Sciences Center, Shreveport, LA, USA*

Introduction

The digestive system has a wide variety of specialized functions that require highly organized and well-regulated vascular beds. While there is considerable heterogeneity of blood flow to different organs in the digestive system, collectively, these tissues account for a large fraction of resting cardiac output (25–30%). The high rate of splanchnic perfusion likely reflects the large mass and significant metabolic needs of this organ system. Blood flow in the splanchnic circulation is, however, dynamic, with increases in flow after ingestion of a meal and reductions in flow during periods of stress that threaten to deprive other organs (e.g., brain, heart) of their normal blood supply. A variety of intrinsic and extrinsic mechanisms allow the splanchnic circulation to respond in a dynamic fashion to changing local tissue requirements and to the overall needs of the body.

In addition to transporting nutrients and oxygen needed to ensure normal health and function of the digestive system, the microcirculation plays a vital role in the movement of water in and out of the interstitial compartment of absorptive (e.g., intestine) and secretory (e.g., pancreas, stomach) organs. Some unique features of the splanchnic microcirculation that optimize the ability to move large amounts of fluid and small solutes between blood and transporting epithelium in these tissues include an unusually high capillary density that increases the surface area for exchange and the presence of fenestrated-type capillaries that provide an enormous pore area for water and solute exchange.

The intrinsic ability of tissues in the digestive system to regulate both blood flow and perfused capillary density allows moment-to-moment adjustments in the delivery of oxygen and exchange of water that ensure efficient organ function. When vascular function is impaired, organ function can be compromised and tissue injury can occur. If blood flow is abnormally decreased, for example, secondary to arterial thrombosis, or increased, as it is in persons with

Gastrointestinal Anatomy and Physiology: The Essentials, First Edition. Edited by John F. Reinus and Douglas Simon.
© 2014 John Wiley & Sons, Ltd. Published 2014 by John Wiley & Sons, Ltd.
www.wiley.com/go/reinus/gastro/anatomy

portal hypertension, resultant dysregulation of the splanchnic circulation will cause pathologic changes in the affected organs. A working knowledge of blood flow regulation in the digestive system and the role of the splanchnic circulation in the transport, metabolic, and motor functions of this system is critical to an understanding of how vascular dysfunction can be an underlying cause of digestive diseases.

Basic principles

Neurohumoral regulation of splanchnic blood flow

Splanchnic blood vessels are richly innervated by both sympathetic and parasympathetic nerve fibers. These fibers release neurotransmitters that alter the tone of vascular smooth muscle (VSM) in arterioles, the major resistance vessels, causing vasodilation or vasoconstriction. Some vasodilator neurotransmitters act directly on VSM receptors to dilate arterioles, while others stimulate nitric oxide (NO) production by vascular endothelium. NO diffuses into underlying VSM to elicit relaxation. Acetylcholine (ACh), vasoactive intestinal peptide (VIP) and substance P are examples of neurotransmitters that are released from parasympathetic nerve fibers, including afferent fibers, to mediate vasodilation via endothelium-dependent NO (Figure 10.1).

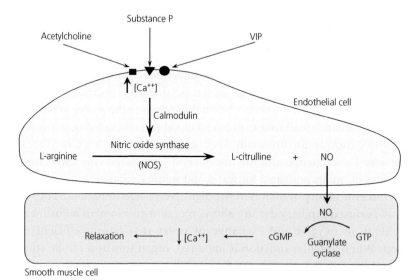

Figure 10.1 NO-mediated relaxation of VSM in splanchnic arterioles. The endothelial cell enzyme NO synthase generates NO following activation with either ACh, substance P, or VIP. The NO diffuses into the underlying smooth muscle cells to activate guanylate cyclase and consequently produce cyclic GMP (cGMP), which lowers intracellular calcium and elicits VSM relaxation.

Sympathetic activation is generally associated with splanchnic vasoconstriction and a reduction in blood flow. Norepinephrine and ATP, potent vasoconstrictors that act directly on VSM to increase arteriolar tone, are the principal mediators of sympathetic vasoconstriction in the splanchnic circulation. While the blood flow reduction elicited by sympathetic activation is profound, this response is not sustained during prolonged sympathetic stimulation, and there is a gradual return of blood flow toward normal despite continued stimulation. This phenomenon, termed "autoregulatory escape," is often attributed to intrinsic metabolic mechanisms that override the neurogenic vasoconstriction.

Splanchnic arterioles are also highly sensitive to circulating vasoconstrictors that are released into blood during periods of whole-body stress, for example, following hemorrhage or trauma. Vasopressin (antidiuretic hormone) and angiotensin II are potent vasoconstrictors that selectively target arterioles in the splanchnic circulation to produce a sustained and prolonged reduction in blood flow. The release of these vasoconstrictors, coupled to the transient yet intense vasoactive effects of sympathetic stimulation, serves to increase total peripheral vascular resistance, maintain blood pressure, and sustain perfusion of vital organs (brain, heart) at the expense of organs in the digestive system.

Intrinsic regulation of blood flow and tissue oxygenation

Organs perfused by the splanchnic circulation typically exhibit only a moderate capacity to regulate blood flow, as compared to heart, brain, and kidney. Pressure-flow autoregulation, that is, the ability of an organ to maintain a relatively constant blood flow when blood pressure is reduced, is not as efficient in splanchnic organs as it is in other vital organs. For example, while a 50% reduction in blood pressure would result in a minimal change in cerebral blood flow, gut blood flow would be reduced by approximately 25%. The fact that neither organ behaves like a passive system (wherein a 50% reduction in flow would be predicted) suggests that the reduction in blood pressure elicits arteriolar dilation and a reduction in vascular resistance, which minimize the fall in blood flow when the perfusion pressure gradient is suddenly reduced. A chemical mediator of arteriolar dilation is adenosine, a potent vasodilator and product of ATP metabolism that accumulates in tissues when blood flow is reduced. Another likely metabolic signal involved in pressure-flow autoregulation and other intrinsic vasoregulatory responses is tissue oxygen tension (tissue pO_2). Reductions in blood flow are associated with a fall in tissue pO_2 because of an imbalance between O_2 delivery and O_2 consumption. Furthermore, the tone of arteriolar VSM is directly correlated with tissue pO_2. Consequently, arteriolar dilation occurs following a hypotension-induced reduction in blood flow. Both tissue pO_2 and adenosine act as mediators of the vasodilation observed in the splanchnic vascular system when oxygen delivery is impaired (e.g., blood flow reduced) or metabolic demand is increased.

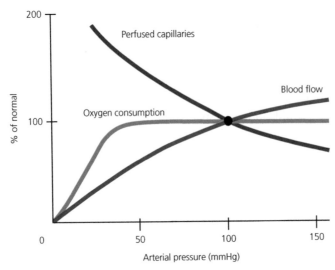

Figure 10.2 Oxygen consumption is better maintained than blood flow in digestive organs when blood pressure is reduced. The recruitment (opening) of more perfused capillaries at low pressures minimizes the distance that oxygen must diffuse between blood and parenchymal cells, thereby facilitating O_2 exchange and maintaining O_2 consumption.

Although blood flow in the splanchnic circulation is not as tightly regulated as it is in other vascular beds, digestive organs are highly efficient in maintaining a level of tissue oxygenation that ensures normal function. As illustrated in Figure 10.2, unlike blood flow, oxygen consumption (VO_2) in splanchnic tissues is maintained at a constant level over a wide range of blood pressures (30–150 mmHg). This precise regulation of VO_2 can be attributed to an increased convective delivery of oxygen due to arteriolar dilation and, more importantly, the recruitment (opening) of more perfused capillaries (only one-third to one-fourth of capillaries are normally open to perfusion) as blood flow is reduced. When more capillaries are open to perfusion at low blood flows, the distance between flowing blood and parenchymal cells is reduced, and tissue pO_2 is maintained at a level that ensures a normal VO_2. Hence, even in the presence of severe hypotension, the combination of arteriolar dilation and capillary recruitment provides a significant margin of safety against tissue hypoxia and tissue injury, affording protection to the splanchnic tissues when they are most vulnerable to ischemic damage.

Regulation of transcapillary fluid exchange

The capillaries of the splanchnic circulation have a high rate of fluid filtration that can be attributed to the water permeability of the fenestrated-type capillaries, the surface area for exchange (high capillary density), and the balance of hydrostatic and oncotic forces exerted across the capillary wall. While the resting capillary filtration rate is high, there is no accumulation of filtered fluid in the interstitial compartment because of the equal rate of interstitial fluid drainage by

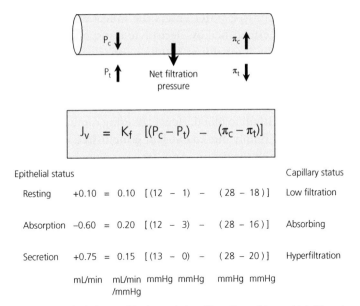

$$J_v = K_f [(P_c - P_t) - (\pi_c - \pi_t)]$$

Epithelial status					Capillary status
Resting	+0.10 = 0.10	[(12 – 1)	–	(28 – 18)]	Low filtration
Absorption	–0.60 = 0.20	[(12 – 3)	–	(28 – 16)]	Absorbing
Secretion	+0.75 = 0.15	[(13 – 0)	–	(28 – 20)]	Hyperfiltration
	mL/min mL/min /mmHg	mmHg mmHg		mmHg mmHg	

Figure 10.3 Changes in the balance of hydrostatic (capillary, P_c, and interstitial, P_t) and oncotic (capillary, π_c, and interstitial, π_t) forces enable capillaries to absorb or filter water (Jv) in accordance with the transport function of epithelial cells in digestive organs. In the absence of epithelial transport (resting state), capillaries filter at a low rate. When water enters the interstitium as a result of epithelial water absorption, the capillaries assume an absorptive phenotype due to the rise in P_t and K_f (a measure of the number of capillaries open to perfusion) and a reduction in π_t. When epithelial cells are stimulated to secrete fluid from interstitium to lumen (gut or duct), interstitial volume falls, which leads to a fall in P_t and an increase in π_t. These changes in interstitial forces are accompanied by increases in P_c and K_f. These changes promote capillary hyperfiltration, which provides the fluid needed for the secretory pump.

the lymphatic system. Large increases in capillary filtration can result when either capillary hydrostatic pressure (e.g., portal hypertension) or vascular permeability (e.g., inflammation) is increased or plasma oncotic pressure is reduced (liver disease). If capillary filtration rate increases beyond the drainage capacity of the lymphatic system, then excess fluid will accumulate in the interstitium (edema) and interstitial fluid pressure will rise, which can compromise blood flow, oxygen exchange, and ultimately organ function. Excess fluid accumulation in the mucosal layer of the gastrointestinal (GI) tract is attenuated because the accompanying elevation in interstitial fluid pressure leads to increased mucosal membrane permeability (epithelial barrier dysfunction) and the consequent filtration of interstitial fluid and protein into the bowel lumen. Inasmuch as the submucosal layer of the GI tract has a low density of terminal lymphatics, this region of the bowel wall more readily exhibits edema formation.

Splanchnic capillaries also play a key role in the water transport function of absorptive and secretory digestive organs (Figure 10.3). In the interdigestive period, intestinal capillaries are in a net-filtering state. Following ingestion of a meal, however, protein-free water enters the mucosal interstitium along a concentration gradient established by electrolyte transport. The accumulation of absorbed water in the interstitium results in an elevated interstitial fluid pressure and a decreased interstitial oncotic pressure (due to dilution of interstitial proteins). With these changes in interstitial forces, the balance of hydrostatic and oncotic pressures across the intestinal capillaries shifts to favor water movement from interstitium to blood. Hence, filtering capillaries are converted to absorbing capillaries simply due to entry of protein-free water from the gut lumen into the mucosal interstitium. Another consequence of elevated interstitial fluid pressure (Pt) during water absorption is increased lymph flow (Pt is the driving force for entry of interstitial fluid into lymphatics). Consequently, absorbed water is promptly removed from the mucosal interstitium by two routes, the capillaries and lymphatics. In secretory organs, electrolyte-coupled water movement occurs in the direction of the gut (or duct) lumen. In this instance, capillary filtration rate must rise to ensure that sufficient fluid is made available to the epithelial lining to perform its secretory function. As fluid moves out of the interstitium and across secretory epithelium, interstitial volume decreases, which results in a decline in Pt and a rise in interstitial oncotic pressure (interstitial proteins are more concentrated following water removal). These changes enhance capillary fluid filtration and diminish the drainage of interstitial fluid through the lymphatics due to the fall in Pt. Arteriolar dilation and resultant increase in capillary pressure, Pc, as well as capillary recruitment also facilitate the delivery of fluid from blood to the secretory pump.

Gastric circulation

Intrinsic regulatory mechanisms adjust gastric blood flow to meet the energy demands of gastric secretion and motility. In addition, gastric blood flow is an important component of the "mucosal defense" system, helping to maintain a barrier against back-diffusion of luminal acid, thereby preventing mucosal damage and ulceration.

Anatomy
Branches of the celiac artery give rise to arterioles in the external muscle layers and the submucosa. Submucosal arterioles branch into capillaries at the bases of glands and pass along the glands to the luminal surface of the mucosa forming capillary networks surrounding the openings of the gastric pits. The mucosal capillaries drain into venules that coalesce to form a dense venous plexus in the submucosa. The submucosal venous drainage penetrates the external muscle layers (where additional venous blood is provided by the muscle microvasculature) and enters the portal vein.

Hemodynamics

The parallel-coupled capillary networks of the gastric muscular layer and the mucosa are under separate control, responding independently to tissue metabolism, other local factors, and extrinsic neural input. At rest (between meals), approximately 75% of total gastric blood flow is distributed to the mucosa, with 25% directed to the muscle layer. This intramural distribution of blood flow is altered when either of the two layers becomes functionally active, that is, when the mucosa is stimulated to produce acid, mucosal blood flow (and its percentage of total flow) preferentially increases.

Regulation of blood flow and oxygenation

Although gastric blood flow autoregulation is modest, gastric oxygen uptake is maintained despite alterations in perfusion pressure. Intrinsic vasoregulatory mechanisms ensure that, as blood flow is reduced, capillary density and oxygen extraction increase sufficiently to maintain tissue oxygenation (Figure 10.2). Gastric oxygen consumption increases in proportion to acid production induced by secretagogues (e.g., gastrin, histamine). In general, there is an increase in gastric blood flow with enhanced secretory activity; however, there are some exceptions. While histamine-induced gastric acid secretion is associated with a local hyperemic response, pentagastrin-induced secretion is not. This is attributed to intrinsic vasoregulatory mechanisms that meet increases in oxygen demand by either increasing oxygen extraction or blood flow or both. Minor reductions in blood flow would not compromise the oxygen delivery necessary to support the increased oxygen demand of acid secretion, since an increase in oxygen extraction (increased capillary density) would make up the deficit. Substantial reductions in gastric blood flow, however, would be associated with decreases in both oxygen delivery and acid secretion; acid secretion would become blood flow limited.

Mucosal defense

The mucus lining covering the gastric surface epithelium offers protection against luminal acid. Capillary transport of parietal cell-derived bicarbonate also plays an important role in protecting the surface epithelium against acid-induced injury and ulceration. Parietal cell H^+ secretion into the lumens of gastric pits is associated with HCO_3^- release into the interstitium. The capillaries surrounding gastric pits transport bicarbonate toward the mucosal surface, where it can diffuse into the interstitial compartment beneath the surface epithelial cells. The latter cells transport bicarbonate into the gastric lumen where it can buffer luminal acid within the mucus layer adjacent to the surface epithelium (Figure 10.4). The vascular contribution to mucosal defense becomes even more important during conditions in which the mucosal barrier to acid back-diffusion is breached. Ingested agents that disrupt mucus production (nonsteroidal anti-inflammatory drugs (NSAIDs), ethanol) or the reflux of mucolytic

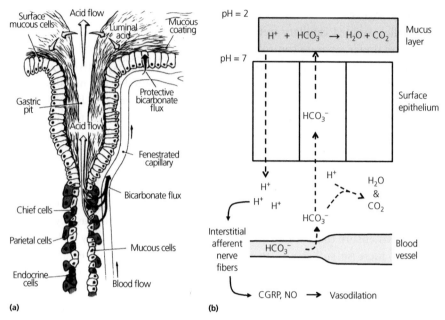

Figure 10.4 (a) Microvascular transport of HCO_3^- from acid-secreting portion of the gastric pit to the surface epithelium. The surface epithelial cells, in turn, transport HCO_3^- into the adherent mucus layer creating a pH gradient decreasing from the epithelium to the gastric lumen. Adapted from *Gastroenterology*, 1984, pp. 866–875. Reproduced with permission from Elsevier. (b) Proposed mechanism by which interstitial H^+ activates a neural reflex that induces a hyperemia to (i) deliver additional HCO_3^- to epithelial cells for transport into the mucus layer and (ii) neutralize the excess H^+ in the interstitium. CGRP, calcitonin gene-related peptide; NO, nitric oxide.

agents (bile salts) are known causes of mucosal injury. Under these conditions, luminal H^+ can enter the interstitium and activate capsaicin receptors on sensory (afferent) neurons. A resultant reflex arc elicits vasodilation through the release of calcitonin gene-related peptide and NO by perivascular neurons (Figure 10.4). Increased mucosal blood flow enhances the delivery of HCO_3^- to surface epithelial cells and neutralizes any H^+ ions that gain access to the mucosal interstitium.

It is generally accepted that severe reductions in mucosal blood flow (e.g., ischemia) render the gastric mucosa vulnerable to the damaging actions of gastric juice and ingested agents, such as ethanol, aspirin, and bacteria (e.g., *Helicobacter pylori*), that may lead to mucosal ulceration and microvascular dysfunction. For example, arteriolar constriction and capillary plugging with either microthrombi or activated leukocytes often accompany the ulceration process and are thought to exacerbate mucosal injury by rendering the tissue ischemic and vulnerable to necrosis. Repair of gastric mucosal ulceration relies on restoration of blood flow and capillary HCO_3^- transport and on growth of new blood vessels (angiogenesis).

Intestinal circulation

Splanchnic blood circulation plays an important role in the support of intestinal functions, including propulsion of chyme and assimilation of ingested nutrients. Intrinsic regulatory mechanisms allow the intestine to adjust the distribution of blood flow between the muscular and mucosal layers in accordance with local metabolic needs. An extensive network of collateral channels within and external to the gut wall also helps to ensure adequate intestinal blood flow.

Anatomy

Blood flow to the intestine is largely derived from vascular arcades arising from the superior mesenteric artery. Arterial vessels are connected by an extensive network of collateral channels found both within the mesentery (extramural) and the bowel wall proper (intramural). The major arterial vessels supplying the mucosa, submucosa, and muscularis emerge from an arterial plexus within the submucosa. The submucosa proper has a relatively sparse capillary network. Arterioles entering the muscle layer branch into capillaries running parallel to muscle fibers. Mucosal villi are supplied by a single arteriole running centrally to the tip where the vessel branches into a fountain-like pattern of capillaries that drain into a centrally located vein. The parallel arrangement, close proximity, and countercurrent flow of blood in villus arterioles and venules suggest that countercurrent shunting of oxygen may occur in intestinal villi. The venous drainage of the mucosa and muscularis empties into large veins within the submucosa. These veins enter the mesentery in parallel to the arterial arcades of the superior mesenteric artery and eventually join the portal vein.

Hemodynamics

Intestinal blood flow accounts for 10–15% of resting cardiac output (500–750 ml/min) in the adult human. In the resting state, approximately 65% of total intestinal blood flow is distributed to the mucosa, 25% to the muscularis, and the remainder to the submucosa. This apportionment of flow within the bowel wall is attributed to the greater metabolic demand of the mucosa. Stimulation of mucosal epithelial transport processes favors increased mucosal perfusion, while enhanced motor activity redistributes blood flow to the muscle layers.

Blood flow regulation

Intrinsic control of intestinal blood flow is mediated by both metabolic and nonmetabolic factors. Ingestion of a meal increases both intestinal blood flow and oxygen consumption. Postprandial hyperemia is confined to that segment of intestine directly exposed to chyme; segments distal to the chyme bolus have normal resting blood flow. Luminal glucose and oleic acid (hydrolytic digestion products) cause intestinal hyperemia: intraluminal glucose does so by stimulating absorption. In contrast, 2-deoxyglucose, which is not absorbed, does not cause hyperemia. Glucose-induced hyperemia is mediated by metabolic factors, such as low tissue pO_2, and adenosine release. The same metabolic factors contribute to oleic acid-induced functional hyperemia, although some of the hyperemia also may be due to mucosal irritation by oleic acid and resultant local release of VIP. The importance of active nutrient transport to postprandial hyperemia is best exemplified by the differential responses of the jejunum and ileum to luminal bile or bile salts. In the jejunum, bile does not cause a hyperemia, while in the ileum, where bile salts are actively transported, luminal bile produces a profound hyperemic response.

Intestinal arterioles are exquisitely sensitive to changes in intravascular pressure and exhibit strong myogenic regulation. This property is attributed to the intrinsic ability of arteriolar smooth muscle to contract in response to stretch. In the presence of a myogenic mechanism, vessel-wall tension (the product of intravascular pressure and vessel radius) is the controlled variable: a sudden rise in intravascular pressure (P) must elicit a reduction in vessel radius (r) in order to maintain a constant vessel-wall tension. Conversely, a reduction in P necessitates an increase in r (vasodilation) in order to maintain a constant T. Myogenic vaso-constriction in the intestine is most evident in the fasting state. In the postprandial state, however, the metabolic demand on the intestine is increased, and intestinal arterioles become more sensitive to metabolic factors (adenosine, tissue pO_2), and myogenic vasoconstriction is overridden by metabolic vasodilation.

Collaterals vessels and ischemia

Occlusion of a major intestinal artery does not necessarily stop or even pro-foundly reduce intestinal blood flow. For example, occlusion of a branch of the superior mesenteric artery in adult animals results in only a 30–50% reduction in intestinal blood flow, which is attributed to an extensive network of intramural and extramural collateral channels. Selective occlusions of the intra-mural and extramural vessels indicate that about two-thirds of total collateral flow is derived from extramural vessels, while the remainder is supplied by intramural collaterals. Poorly developed collaterals, coupled with impaired pressure-flow autoregulation, appear to render the neonatal intestine more susceptible to ischemia.

Reperfusion of the ischemic intestine exacerbates microvascular dysfunction and tissue injury caused by ischemia. Reperfusion-induced intestinal pathology is comparable to that observed during an intense inflammatory response. Reintroduction of oxygen with reperfusion results in local formation of oxygen radicals, which in turn initiates a series of events that promote recruitment and activation of neutrophils. Extravasated neutrophils release a variety of prote-ases and reactive oxygen metabolites that mediate the mucosal dysfunction and epithelial necrosis induced by ischemia and reperfusion.

Pancreatic circulation

Production of pancreatic juice requires (i) oxygen delivery to meet the metabolic demands of electrolyte transport and (ii) fluid transport from blood into pancreatic ducts. The pancreatic circulation is regulated to meet both the oxygen and fluid demands of pancreatic exocrine secretion. The existence of a portal circulation between the endocrine and exocrine portions of the gland allows hormones secreted by islet cells to modulate acinar and ductal function.

Anatomy

The pancreas is supplied by arterial blood from two sources: the superior pancreaticoduodenal artery (derived from the celiac artery) and the inferior pancreaticoduodenal artery (derived from the superior mesenteric artery). The existence of extrapancreatic collaterals implies that, as in the intestine, pancreatic blood flow will not be substantially compromised by occlusion of one of the supplying arteries. Within the pancreas, arterioles perfuse the three functional gland components: acini, ducts, and islets. Blood from all three plexi drains into either the splenic vein or the superior mesenteric vein, which ultimately empties into the portal vein.

There is also an extensive portal circulation within the pancreas. Blood vessels from the capillary plexi within the islets of Langerhans join the acinar and ductal plexi prior to draining into the venous system. The functional significance of this intrapancreatic portal circulation is that hormones secreted by the islets reach the exocrine portion of the gland (the acini and ducts) in very high concentrations. Virtually all of the peptide hormones secreted by the islets (especially insulin) influence pancreatic secretion.

Blood flow regulation

Metabolic factors appear to be the major determinants of blood flow and tissue oxygenation in the resting pancreas. Reduced blood flow (caused by a decrease in arterial, or an increase in venous, pressure) increases oxygen extraction so that net oxygen uptake is maintained. Enhanced secretory activity induced by a meal or secretagogues results in a two- to threefold increase in pancreatic blood flow. A portion of this functional hyperemia is attributed to the increased metabolic demand of active electrolyte transport by pancreatic acini and ducts. The hyperemic response also ensures the delivery of water required by the secretory process. The kallikrein–kinin system, cholinergic and purinergic neurotransmitters, and GI hormones (cholecystokinin and secretin) have all been implicated in the vasodilation associated with enhanced pancreatic secretory activity. Arteriolar dilation elevates pancreatic capillary hydrostatic pressure, which drives fluid across the capillaries into the interstitial spaces surrounding the transporting epithelium (Figure 10.3). The importance of these vascular adjustments to enhanced pancreatic secretion is underscored by the fact that during periods of maximal stimulation, the pancreas can secrete its weight in juice in less than 30 min.

Hepatic circulation

The hepatic circulation is unique in several ways: the liver is perfused by both arterial and portal venous afferent vessels that combine to deliver a large fraction (25%) of cardiac output. The acinar arrangement of the hepatic microvasculature creates a series of microenvironments within the organ that imparts a significant spatial restriction to specific biosynthetic, biotransformation, and detoxification functions of the liver.

Anatomy

The liver receives fully oxygenated blood from the high-pressure, high-resistance hepatic artery, while partially oxygenated blood comes from the low-pressure, low-resistance portal vein (Chapter 10). These vessels give rise to numerous smaller vessels within the liver, called hepatic arterioles and terminal portal venules, which perfuse a small mass of parenchyma called the liver acinus. Mixed arterial and venous blood enters the hepatic sinusoids, which constitute the capillary network of the liver. The sinusoidal capillaries are highly permeable to water and plasma proteins, explaining the high protein concentration of hepatic interstitial fluid and lymph. The sinusoids radiate toward the periphery of the acinus, where they connect with the terminal hepatic venules and ultimately into progressively larger branches of hepatic veins and the inferior vena cava.

Hemodynamics

The portal vein supplies the liver with 70–75% of its blood, while the hepatic artery provides the remaining 25–30%. Because of the higher oxygen content of arterial blood, the hepatic artery and portal vein contribute roughly equal amounts of oxygen to the liver in the fasting state. The mean blood pressure in the hepatic artery is about 90 mmHg and that in the portal vein about 10 mmHg, with a sinusoidal capillary pressure of 2–3 mmHg. The low pressure within these highly permeable capillaries serves to minimize excessive loss of fluid and protein into the liver interstitium and subsequent leakage of this plasma filtrate into the peritoneal cavity (ascites fluid).

The liver also represents the most important blood reservoir in man, containing about 15% of the total blood volume. Hepatic blood volume can nearly double when right atrial pressure is elevated. The capacitance function of the liver plays an important role during bleeding. After moderate blood loss, activated sympathetic nerves constrict the hepatic venules and expel enough blood to compensate for as much as 25% of lost volume.

Blood flow regulation

A decrease in portal venous blood flow causes a reduction in hepatic arterial resistance, while an increase in portal venous flow results in hepatic arterial constriction. This reciprocal relationship between hepatic arterial and portal venous blood flows tends to maintain a relatively constant total blood flow through the liver. Hepatic arterioles, however, cannot fully compensate for severe reductions in portal venous inflow volume. Nonetheless, the liver maintains a constant level of oxygen consumption because the extraction of oxygen from hepatic blood is very efficient. The small distance for oxygen diffusion between blood and hepatocytes accounts for this highly efficient oxygen extraction. Hepatic blood flow increases following ingestion of a meal, largely due to increased flow in the portal vein.

Portal hypertension

Chronic portal hypertension (CPH) usually is associated with increased resistance to portal venous inflow (intrahepatic portal hypertension). The resultant increase in portal pressure promotes shunting of blood from the splanchnic to the systemic circulation through collateral vessels (both preexisting and induced) that bypass the liver. Compensatory decompression of the portal vein by shunting of blood away from the liver tends to be neutralized by vasodilation of splanchnic blood vessels and also of vessels in other regional vascular beds. Vasodilation in response to portal hypertension has been attributed to induction of vasodilatory substances (e.g., NO, vascular endothelial growth factor) and also to an increased resistance of splanchnic vasculature to endogenous vasoconstrictors (e.g., norepinephrine). Altered vasodilator and vasoconstrictor responses in CPH have been linked to abnormalities in NO production by arteriolar endothelium and NO responsiveness by arteriolar VSM. As shown in Figure 10.5, the

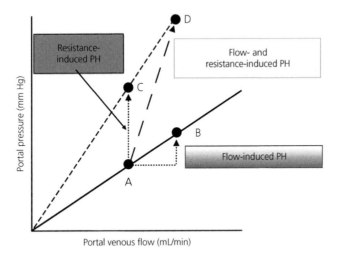

Figure 10.5 The dependency of portal pressure on portal blood flow when portal vascular resistance is normal (solid line) or increased (broken line). Increasing blood flow leads to an increased portal pressure when vascular resistance is either normal (point A to point B) or elevated (point C to point D). When both blood flow and vascular resistance are increased (e.g., portal hypertension), a more substantial increase in portal pressure occurs (point A to point D).

relationship between portal venous pressure and portal flow predicts that the combination of increased vascular resistance and increased portal blood flow produces a more substantial elevation of portal pressure than predicted by either factor (flow and resistance) alone. Therapies for portal hypertension have focused on reducing either the hyperdynamic circulation (e.g., vasopressin) or the increased intrahepatic resistance (e.g., angiotensin receptor blockers).

A predictable complication of portal hypertension is microvascular dysfunction in upstream organs, such as the stomach (portal hypertensive gastropathy (PHG)), intestine (portal hypertensive enteropathy), and colon (portal hypertensive colonopathy). PHG, the best documented complication, is characterized by congested mucosal capillaries, edema, and reduced mucosal blood flow but little bleeding or ulceration. These responses render the gastric mucosa more susceptible to injury by luminal irritants (NSAIDs, ethanol, or bile salts). Furthermore, the stomach cannot mount a hyperemic response when the mucosa is exposed by these luminal irritants.

Multiple choice questions

1 Splanchnic blood flow:
   A Is unchanged after ingestion of a meal
   B Is higher in the muscularis than mucosal layers
   C Exhibits a stronger myogenic response in the fed than fasted state
   D Escapes from the vasoconstrictor influence of sympathetic activation
   E Exhibits nearly perfect pressure-flow autoregulation
2 Which of the following is *least* likely to elicit a reduction in splanchnic blood flow?
   A Severe exercise
   B Hemorrhage
   C Massive sympathoadrenal discharge
   D Heart failure
   E Chronic portal hypertension
3 An increase in gastric mucosal blood flow during acid secretion protects the mucosa from damage by:
   A Providing fluid for acid secretion
   B Removing urea from the interstitium
   C Preventing edema formation
   D Delivering bicarbonate to surface epithelial cells
   E Enhancing mucus secretion
4 The microvascular responses to enhanced pancreatic secretion include:
   A A decrease in protein leakage
   B A decrease in capillary pressure
   C Enhanced fluid filtration
   D Vasoconstriction
   E Removal of bicarbonate from the interstitium
5 The major determinant of mesenteric blood flow is:
   A Arterial pressure
   B Venous pressure
   C Vascular resistance

6 Endothelium-dependent vasodilation results from which of the following factors:

A Endothelin

B Nitric oxide

C Acetylcholine

D Calcitonin gene-related peptide

Further Reading

Gannon, B. (1984) Mucosal microvascular architecture of the funds and body of human stomach. *Gastroenterology*, **86**, 866–875.

Granger, D.N., Barrowman, J.A. and Kvietys, P.R. (1985) *Clinical Gastrointestinal Physiology*, WB Saunders, Philadelphia.

Holzer, P. (2007) Role of visceral afferent neurons in mucosal inflammation and defense. *Current Opinion in Pharmacology*, **7**, 563–569.

Holzer, P. (2012) Neural regulation of gastrointestinal blood flow, in *Physiology of the Gastrointestinal Tract*, 5th edn (eds L.R. Johnson), Elsevier-Academic Press, London, pp. 817–845.

Kvietys, P. (2010) The gastrointestinal circulation, in *Colloquium Series in Integrated Systems Physiology: From Molecule to Function* (eds D.N. Granger and J.P. Granger), Morgan & Claypool Life Sciences, San Rafael.

Kvietys, P.R., Granger, D.N. and Harper, S.L. (1989) Circulation of the pancreas and salivary glands, in *Handbook of Physiology*. Section 6. *The Gastrointestinal System*. Vol **1** *Motility and Circulation*, Part 2, pp. 1565–1595.

Lautt, W.W. (2010) Hepatic circulation: physiology & pathophysiology, in *Colloquium Series in Integrated Systems Physiology: From Molecule to Function* (eds D.N. Granger and J.P. Granger), Morgan & Claypool Life Sciences, San Rafael.

Nowicki, P.T., Crissinger, K.D. and Granger, D.N. (2009) Gastrointestinal blood flow, in *Textbook of Gastroenterology* 5th edn (ed. T. Yamada) Williams and Wilkins, Lippincott, Vol. **1**, pp. 498–520.

Perini, R.F., Camara, P.R.S. and Ferraz, J.G.P. (2009) Pathogenesis of portal hypertensive gastropathy: translating basic research into clinical practice. *Nature Reviews Gastroenterology and Hepatology*, **6**, 150–158.

Wallace, J.L. and Granger, D.N. (1996) The cellular and molecular basis of gastric mucosal defense. *FASEB Journal*, **10**, 731–740.

Answers

1 D

2 E

3 D

4 C

5 C

6 B

CHAPTER 11

Composition and circulation of the bile

Allan W. Wolkoff

Division of Gastroenterology and Liver Diseases, Marion Bessin Liver Research Center, Albert Einstein College of Medicine and Montefiore Medical Center, Bronx, NY, USA

Introduction

Bile is an essential fluid that delivers bile acids, lipids, and metabolites to the intestine. In many ways, one can consider the liver and bile as being analogous to the kidney and urine. It has been estimated that the normal adult produces about 0.5 l of bile each day. Like urine, bile is primarily composed of water. Eighty percent of bile by weight is water, and the remainder consists of bile acids, phospholipids, cholesterol, bile pigments, and electrolytes. The solid components of bile have major physiologic importance with respect to processes such as intestinal absorption and excretion.

Mechanism of bile formation

Bile is formed by a complex mechanism that requires hepatocyte secretion of bile acids and other solutes, such as glutathione (GSH) and bicarbonate, and secretion of bicarbonate by bile ductular cells. Water passively follows these constituents into the bile canaliculi and ducts, creating bile flow [1, 2]. The components of bile formation have been termed (i) bile acid dependent, (ii) bile acid independent, and (iii) ductular. Under baseline conditions, most bile formation results from hepatocyte excretion of bile acids into the bile canaliculus. As discussed in the succeeding text, bile acids are synthesized in hepatocytes from cholesterol, conjugated with glycine or taurine, and pumped across the bile canaliculus into the biliary tree [3]. The bile salt export pump (BSEP) is ATP dependent and resides on the bile canalicular plasma membrane. It is officially designated as the ATP-binding cassette, subfamily B, member 11 (ABCB11), but it is still usually referred to as BSEP. Although excretion of bile acids with accompanying water results in a major portion of bile formation (bile acid-dependent

Gastrointestinal Anatomy and Physiology: The Essentials, First Edition. Edited by John F. Reinus and Douglas Simon.
© 2014 John Wiley & Sons, Ltd. Published 2014 by John Wiley & Sons, Ltd.
www.wiley.com/go/reinus/gastro/anatomy

bile flow), excretion of GSH and bicarbonate by other transport proteins on the hepatocyte canalicular membrane is responsible for a potentially important fraction of bile formation (bile acid-independent bile flow) [2].

Chemistry of bile acids

Bile acids are derivatives of cholesterol (Figure 11.1) [4, 5]. They are synthesized by hepatocytes and can be modified by bacteria as they transit the intestine. The hepatocyte synthesizes two primary bile acids: cholic and chenodeoxycholic acid. The secondary bile acids, deoxycholic, taurocholic, lithocholic, and ursodeoxy-cholic acid, are formed from the primary bile acids by actions of bacterial enzymes in the intestinal lumen. Secondary bile acids can be absorbed across the intestinal mucosa, entering the portal circulation from which they can be extracted by hepatocytes. Lithocholic acid is the least soluble of these compounds, and consequently, most gets excreted in the stool, although a small fraction can be found in the bile acid pool. Primary and secondary bile acids within hepatocytes are conjugated with the amino acids glycine or taurine (Figure 11.2). This makes them more water soluble (hydrophilic) at physiologic pH, reducing their pKa from approximately 5.0 to 4.0 (glycine conjugates) and 2.0 (taurine conjugates). This increased hydrophilicity reduces their ability to cross the cell membrane lipid bilayer. Consequently, conjugated bile acids require the presence of specific transport proteins to be taken up or excreted by cells (Figure 11.3).

Bile acid transport and the enterohepatic circulation

Uptake of bile acids by hepatocytes

Bile acids are required for micelle formation in the intestine. Their efficient reabsorption into the portal circulation and uptake by hepatocytes conserves bile acids, minimizing fecal loss and the energy cost of synthesis. It is the small amount of bile acids that are lost in stool, however, that represents the major pathway by which the body eliminates cholesterol. The high efficiency of entero-hepatic cycling of bile acids results in daily fecal loss of only approximately 5% of the total bile acid pool. In the normal steady-state situation, that means that only approximately 5% of the bile acid pool needs to be synthesized each day. This important mechanism is mediated by a number of specific transporters in the hepatocyte and small intestine [6] (Figure 11.3). Previous studies have shown that approximately 75% of hepatocyte uptake of conjugated bile acids is Na^+ dependent; two Na^+ ions are taken up with each bile acid molecule. The remainder of bile acid uptake is mediated by Na^+-independent mechanisms. A transport protein that can mediate Na^+-dependent bile acid transport

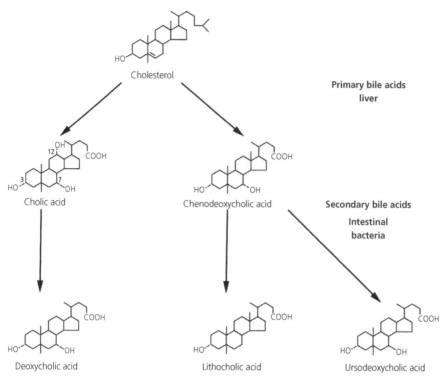

Figure 11.1 Synthesis of bile acids: cholic and chenodeoxycholic acids are synthesized in hepatocytes from cholesterol and are known as primary bile acids. They differ from cholesterol through shortening of the side chain and hydroxylation patterns of the ring structure. The 3-OH group of cholesterol is in the β configuration, as indicated by a solid line, and becomes epimerized to the α configuration, indicated by a dashed line, during the biosynthetic process. The α and β designations refer to whether the hydroxyl group is below or above the plane of the steroid ring, respectively. Hydroxylation at the 7 and 12 positions results in formation of cholic acid, while addition of a hydroxyl group at the 7 position alone in addition to that at the 3 position results in formation of chenodeoxycholic acid. All of these hydroxyl groups are in the α configuration. Within the intestine, there are bacteria that 7-dehydroxylate the primary bile acids cholic and chenodeoxycholic acids resulting in formation of the secondary bile acids deoxycholic and lithocholic acids, respectively. In addition, a small amount of ursodeoxycholic acid is formed from chenodeoxycholic acid by epimerization of the 7-α hydroxyl group to 7-β. These bile acids can be absorbed from the intestine and added to the bile acid pool, although the poor aqueous solubility of lithocholic acid limits its availability.

$$\text{BA}-\overset{\overset{\displaystyle O}{\|}}{C}-\underset{\underset{\displaystyle H}{|}}{N}-CH_2COO^- \qquad \textbf{Glycine}$$

$$\text{BA}-\overset{\overset{\displaystyle O}{\|}}{C}-\underset{\underset{\displaystyle H}{|}}{N}-(CH_2)_2SO_2O^- \qquad \textbf{Taurine}$$

Figure 11.2 Conjugation of bile acids: within the hepatocyte, all bile acids are conjugated with the amino acids glycine or taurine at the carboxyl side chain. In humans, glycine is the predominant conjugate. Conjugation serves to increase the solubility of the bile acids at physiologic pH. Although most conjugated bile acids are reabsorbed from the small intestine, the small amount that reaches the colon can be deconjugated by bacteria and reabsorbed passively through the intestinal lumen into the portal circulation. They can then be extracted by hepatocytes and reconjugated.

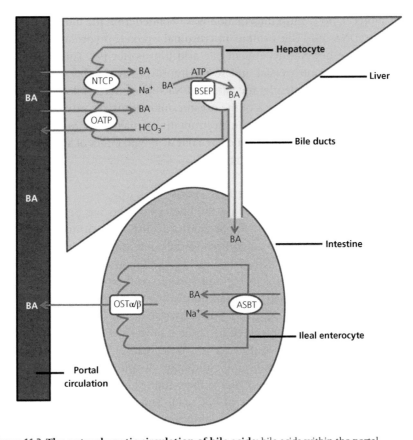

Figure 11.3 The enterohepatic circulation of bile acids: bile acids within the portal circulation are taken up avidly by hepatocytes via the NTCP that mediates their predominant Na^+-dependent uptake or an organic anion transport protein (OATP) that mediates their Na^+-independent uptake in exchange for an anion such as HCO_3^-. Bile acids are subsequently pumped out of the hepatocyte into bile by an ATP-dependent pump termed BSEP. Bile acids in bile flow into the small intestine where they are efficiently recovered. The major transporters for bile acid recovery are located in the ileal enterocyte of the terminal ileum. They are taken up into the cell by a Na^+-dependent protein called the ASBT that resides on the brush border membrane of the enterocytes. This transporter is related to but distinct from NTCP, the Na^+-dependent hepatocyte bile acid transporter. Bile acids within the ileal enterocytes are exported into the portal circulation by a heteromeric protein termed OST that is composed of two subunits, OST-α and OST-β. The cycle can then repeat. The enterohepatic circulation of bile acids is highly efficient recovering approximately 95% per day of bile acids that are secreted into the intestine.

has been identified using molecular biology tools [6, 7]. This protein, named Na^+–taurocholate cotransport protein (NTCP), is primarily expressed on the hepatocyte sinusoidal plasma membrane. Although it can mediate high affinity bile acid transport when studied *in vitro* in cell lines transfected with this transporter, its role *in vivo* has not been confirmed. There are no NTCP knockout animal models. Although polymorphisms that perturb NTCP-mediated transport *in vitro* have been described in samples of DNA obtained from anonymous human subjects, no clinical information was obtained from the individuals who donated the DNA [8]. The protein microsomal epoxide hydrolase has been proposed as another Na^+-dependent bile acid transporter [9]. This suggestion, however, remains controversial and so far unproven. A number of candidate transport proteins are potential mediators of Na^+-independent bile acid uptake. Chief among these are members of the organic anion transport protein family of transporters. These proteins mediate electroneutral uptake, and most appear to couple uptake of an organic anion such as a bile acid with efflux of another anion such as HCO_3^- out of the cell [10, 11].

Excretion of bile acids by hepatocytes

The concentration of bile acids within the bile canaliculus has been estimated to be approximately 1000 times that of their concentration within the hepatocyte. This implies that energy is required for bile acid transport into the canaliculus. Several studies indicated that bile acid excretion into the bile canaliculus requires ATP as the energy source, and further studies identified the ATP-dependent excretory pump as a protein that had been previously named sister of P-glycoprotein (SPGP) [12]. SPGP was known to be concentrated at the bile canalicular membrane and received its name due to its close amino acid similarity to P-glycoprotein, a multidrug resistance protein that was found to protect cancer cells from chemotherapeutic agents by pumping them out of the cell. Subsequently, studies were performed that showed that SPGP could mediate ATP-dependent transport of bile acids and that its absence resulted in severe cholestatic syndromes, including progressive familial intrahepatic cholestasis type-2 (PFIC2), in which bile acid content of bile was very low, while very high levels of bile acids accumulated in the circulation. Based on this information, the name, SPGP, was changed to BSEP, and its official name was given as ABCB11 by an international nomenclature committee. BSEP mutations that result in partial loss of activity are responsible, in part, for the syndrome of benign recurrent intrahepatic cholestasis (BRIC). Patients with BRIC may also have mutations of the genes encoding FIC1, which is thought to be an aminophospholipid transporter that maintains phospholipid content of the inner leaflet of the plasma membrane, serving in some way to protect the bile canalicular membrane from the detergent effects of bile acids [13].

Transport of bile acids by intestinal epithelial cells

As noted earlier, intestinal absorption of bile acids is a highly efficient process that recovers approximately 95% of bile acids secreted into the intestine. Although there is a small amount of passive absorption of bile acids in the proximal small intestine, the major location of bile acid absorption is the distal ileum, which is the site of an active bile acid transport mechanism. The importance of the distal ileum in bile acid homeostasis is apparent in patients who develop large-scale bile acid malabsorption and consequent maldigestion following ileal resection. Studies have revealed that active ileal transport of bile acids is mediated by a protein named the apical sodium bile acid transporter (ASBT), which is located on the brush border membrane of enterocytes. This transporter is related to but distinct from NTCP, the Na^+-dependent hepatocyte bile acid transporter. Its physiologic importance has been appreciated from study of patients with primary bile acid malabsorption in which loss-of-function mutations in the gene encoding ASBT have been documented [14, 15]. The ileal enterocyte also has a mechanism to export intracellular bile acids into the portal circulation. This is mediated by a heteromeric protein termed organic solute transporter (OST) that is composed of two subunits, OST-α and OST-β [16–18].

Functions of bile acids

Approximately 70% of the solid constituents of bile are bile acids. They are critically important to formation of mixed micelles, complexing with the two other major components of bile, phospholipids and cholesterol. Phospholipids are excreted into bile by the multidrug resistance-3 protein (MDR3), also known as ATP-binding cassette, subfamily B, member 4 (ABCB4), which is located at the bile canalicular membrane. Persons with mutations of MDR3 have progressive familial intrahepatic cholestasis type-3 (PFIC3), characterized by very low concentrations of phospholipids in bile. As a result, their bile

Table 11.1 Comparison of familial disorders of hepatocyte bile acid transport and homeostasis.

	Age at presentation	Symptoms	Development	GGT	Protein defect
PFIC syndromes					
PFIC1 (Byler's disease)	Childhood	Severe cholestatic symptoms	Retarded growth	Normal	FIC1 functionally absent
PFIC2	Childhood	Severe cholestatic symptoms	Retarded growth	Normal	BSEP functionally absent
PFIC3	Variable	Severe cholestatic symptoms	Usually normal development	Elevated	MDR3 functionally absent
BRIC syndromes					
BRIC1	Variable	Episodic cholestasis	Normal	Normal	FIC1 reduced activity
BRIC2	Variable	Episodic cholestasis	Normal	Normal	BSEP reduced activity

canaliculi and bile ducts are exposed to high levels of bile acids that act as detergents, solubilizing cell membranes. Affected individuals develop symptomatic cholestasis later in life as a consequence of liver and bile duct injury [19]. They also have impaired formation of mixed micelles.

Mixed-micelle formation is necessary for intestinal absorption of lipophilic dietary components and to keep biliary cholesterol in solution. Bile acids have both hydrophilic and hydrophobic domains (amphiphilic). They are soluble in aqueous solution, and when their concentration exceeds what has been termed the critical micellar concentration, they form micelles in which the interior is hydrophobic, while the exterior is hydrophilic. These micelles can solubilize phospholipids, forming a mixed micelle that facilitates incorporation of cholesterol, which is otherwise insoluble in water. This mixed micelle composed of bile acids, phospholipids, and cholesterol serves to keep cholesterol in solution in bile. The ratio of these three micellar components is important, and perturbation of their equilibrium can result in cholesterol precipitation and formation of cholesterol gallstones [20].

Multiple choice questions

1 Which one of the following statements about bile acids is true?
   A They are synthesized from heme in reticuloendothelial cells.
   B They are synthesized from cholesterol in hepatocytes.
   C They are secreted in the intestine and largely excreted in the stool.
   D Their conjugation with glucuronic acid is required for excretion into bile.
   E Their excretion into bile does not require energy.

2 A 50-year-old woman has right-sided abdominal pain and is found to have gallstones. A sample of bile is taken for analysis during surgery in which her gallbladder was removed. Analysis of the gallstone showed that it did not contain bilirubin. Which one of the following statements is true?
   A Bile acid crystals will be seen when the bile is examined under a microscope.
   B Phospholipid and cholesterol content of her bile will be much higher than normal.
   C Cholesterol will be the major component of the gallstone.
   D She has a disorder in which phospholipids cannot be taken up by hepatocytes.
   E Her bile will be clear due to inability to excrete bilirubin.

3 A 3-month-old baby girl has a mutation in the bile salt excretory protein (BSEP) gene that results in no expression of this protein. Which of the following is a clinical consequence of this finding?
   A She will have periodic episodes of cholestasis.
   B She will develop normally although she may be jaundiced.
   C Bile acid levels in the circulation will be low.
   D Bile acid levels in the circulation will be elevated.
   E Her parents will both have the same symptoms as she as.

4 Which of the following is true concerning bile?
   A Formation of bile is due in part to excretion of bilirubin by the liver cell.
   B Conjugation of bile acids with glucuronic acid is necessary for their excretion into bile.
   C Formation of the secondary bile acids occurs in the endoplasmic reticulum of the liver cell.

 D Formation of bile is due in part to excretion of bile acids by the liver cell.

 E Conversion of bilirubin to bile acids regulates bile flow.

5 Secondary bile acids are formed:

 A In the liver from cholesterol

 B By the conjugation of bile salts with taurine or glycine

 C Both

 D Neither

6 The rate-limiting step for enterohepatic cycling of bile salts is:

 A Canalicular secretion of bile salts

 B Contraction of the gallbladder following a meal

 C Intestinal motility

 D Ileal uptake of bile salts

References

1 Marinelli, R.A., Lehmann, G.L., Soria, L.R. and Marchissio, M.J. (2011) Hepatocyte aquaporins in bile formation and cholestasis. *Frontiers in Bioscience*, **16**, 2642–2652.

2 Wagner, M., Zollner, G. and Trauner, M. (2009) New molecular insights into the mechanisms of cholestasis. *Journal of Hepatology*, **51**, 565–580.

3 Russell, D.W. (2003) The enzymes, regulation, and genetics of bile acid synthesis. *Annual Review of Medicine*, **72**, 137–174.

4 Heubi, J.E., Setchell, K.D. and Bove, K.E. (2007) Inborn errors of bile acid metabolism. *Seminars in Liver Disease*, **27**, 282–294.

5 Chiang, J.Y. (2004) Regulation of bile acid synthesis: pathways, nuclear receptors, and mechanisms. *Journal of Hepatology*, **40**, 539–551.

6 Kosters, A. and Karpen, S.J. (2008) Bile acid transporters in health and disease. *Xenobiotica*, **38**, 1043–1071.

7 Meier, P.J. and Stieger, B. (2002) Bile salt transporters. *Annual Review of Physiology*, **64**, 635–661.

8 Ho, R.H., Leake, B.F., Roberts, R.L. *et al.* (2004) Ethnicity-dependent polymorphism in Na$^+$–taurocholate cotransporting polypeptide (SLC10A1) reveals a domain critical for bile acid substrate recognition. *Journal of Molecular Medicine*, **279**, 7213–7222.

9 von Dippe, P., Amoui, M., Stellwagen, R.H. and Levy, D. (1996) The functional expression of sodium-dependent bile acid transport in Madin-Darby canine kidney cells transfected with the cDNA for microsomal epoxide hydrolase. *Journal of Molecular Medicine*, **271**, 18176–18180.

10 Wolkoff, A.W. and Cohen, D.E. (2003) Bile acid regulation of hepatic physiology: I. Hepatocyte transport of bile acids. *American Journal of Physiology: Gastrointestinal and Liver Physiology*, **284**, G175–G179.

11 Choi, J.H., Murray, J.W. and Wolkoff, A.W. (2011) PDZK1 binding and serine phosphorylation regulate subcellular trafficking of organic anion transport protein 1a1. *American Journal of Physiology: Gastrointestinal and Liver Physiology*, **300**, G384–G393.

12 Stieger, B., Meier, Y. and Meier, P.J. (2007) The bile salt export pump. *Pflügers Archiv - European Journal of Physiology*, **453**, 611–620.

13 Paulusma, C.C., Groen, A., Kunne, C.*et al.* (2006) Atp8b1 deficiency in mice reduces resistance of the canalicular membrane to hydrophobic bile salts and impairs bile salt transport. *Hepatology*, **44**, 195–204.

14 Wong, M.H., Oelkers, P. and Dawson, P.A. (1995) Identification of a mutation in the ileal sodium-dependent bile acid transporter gene that abolishes transport activity. *Journal of Molecular Medicine*, **270**, 27228–27234.

15 Oelkers, P., Kirby, L.C., Heubi, J.E. and Dawson, P.A. (1997) Primary bile acid malabsorption caused by mutations in the ileal sodium-dependent bile acid transporter gene (SLC10A2). *Journal of Clinical Investigation,* **99**, 1880–1887.

16 Rao, A., Haywood, J., Craddock, A.L. *et al.* (2008) The organic solute transporter alpha-beta, Ostalpha-Ostbeta, is essential for intestinal bile acid transport and homeostasis. *Proceedings of the National Academy of Sciences of the United States of America,* **105**, 3891–3896.

17 Ballatori, N., Li, N., Fang, F. *et al.* (2009) OST alpha-OST beta: a key membrane transporter of bile acids and conjugated steroids. *Frontiers in Bioscience,* **14**, 2829–2844.

18 Dawson, P.A., Hubbert, M.L. and Rao, A. (2010) Getting the mOST from OST: role of organic solute transporter, OSTalpha-OSTbeta, in bile acid and steroid metabolism. *Biochimica et Biophysica Acta,* **1801**, 994–1004.

19 Davit-Spraul, A., Gonzales, E., Baussan, C.and Jacquemin, E. (2010) The spectrum of liver diseases related to ABCB4 gene mutations: pathophysiology and clinical aspects. *Seminars in Liver Disease,* **30**, 134–146.

20 Wang, D.Q., Cohen, D.E. and Carey, M.C. (2009) Biliary lipids and cholesterol gallstone disease. *The Journal of Lipid Research,* **50** (Suppl), S406–S411.

Answers

1 B
2 C
3 D
4 D
5 D
6 A

CHAPTER 12

Bilirubin metabolism

Allan W. Wolkoff

Division of Gastroenterology and Liver Diseases, Marion Bessin Liver Research Center, Albert Einstein College of Medicine and Montefiore Medical Center, Bronx, NY, USA

Sources of bilirubin

Bilirubin is a degradation product of heme (Figure 12.1). Senescent red blood cells are the source of most serum bilirubin, but bilirubin is also produced as a result of degradation of other heme proteins, such as cytochromes and myoglobin [1].

The first step in bilirubin production is opening of the tetrapyrollic heme ring at its α-methene bridge. This process is catalyzed by the enzyme heme oxygenase, which forms the green compound, biliverdin, while releasing an atom of iron and a molecule of carbon monoxide (CO). Degradation of heme is the only endogenous source of CO, and CO production has been used as a measure of bilirubin production in research studies. Recent investigations have indicated that CO may serve as an important second messenger and vasomotor regulator [2]. Biliverdin is water soluble and represents the major bile pigment in amphibia, fish, and birds. In mammals, however, biliverdin is converted to the yellow compound bilirubin, a process catalyzed by the enzyme biliverdin reductase (Figure 12.1). The reason for this extra step in mammalian heme degradation is not known but has been attributed by some to the fact that biliverdin does not cross the placenta, while the placenta has a transport mechanism to remove bilirubin from the fetal circulation and deliver it to the maternal circulation from which it is removed by the liver.

Although senescent red blood cells are degraded primarily in the spleen, heme production can occur in reticuloendothelial cells throughout the body as well as in cells such as hepatocytes and renal tubular cells that have high turnover of heme-containing proteins. Hyperbilirubinemia following a large tissue extravasation of blood such as might occur after trauma or pulmonary embolus has been described and is attributed to increased formation of bilirubin in these tissues. It should be pointed out that the common "black and blue mark" is due to heme

Gastrointestinal Anatomy and Physiology: The Essentials, First Edition. Edited by John F. Reinus and Douglas Simon.
© 2014 John Wiley & Sons, Ltd. Published 2014 by John Wiley & Sons, Ltd.
www.wiley.com/go/reinus/gastro/anatomy

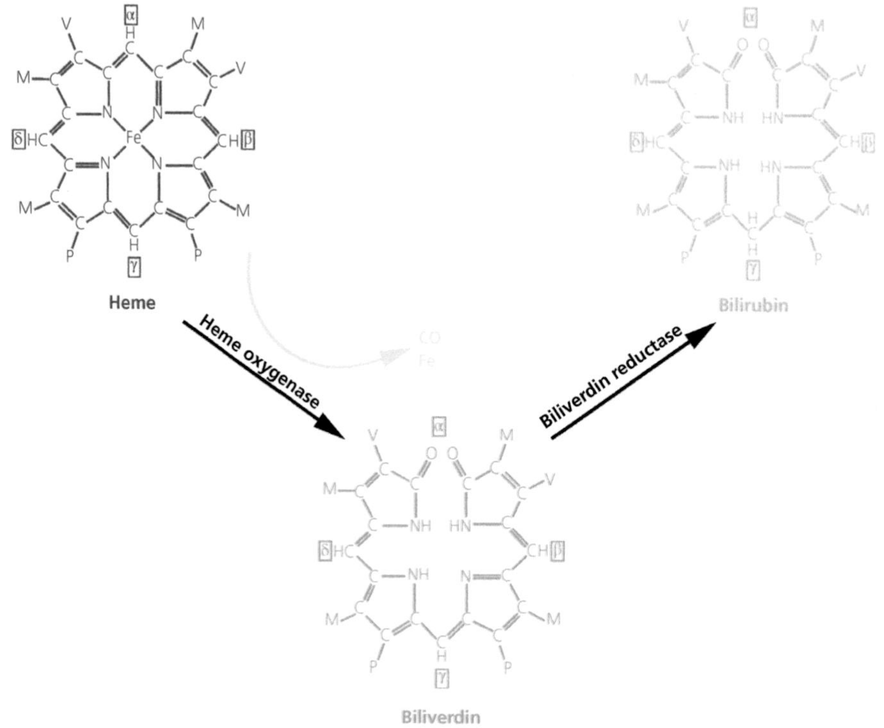

Figure 12.1 Pathway of bilirubin formation from heme: bilirubin is a degradation product of heme that is released from senescent red blood cells as well as other heme proteins such as cytochromes. The first step in this process is opening of the tetrapyrrollic heme ring at its α-methene bridge. This process is catalyzed by the enzyme heme oxygenase and results in release of an atom of iron and a molecule of carbon monoxide (CO) and formation of the green compound, biliverdin. This reaction is the only endogenous source of CO, a gas that may have important biological signal transduction effects. Biliverdin is converted to the yellow compound bilirubin, catalyzed by the enzyme biliverdin reductase.

catabolism and bilirubin formation. Initially, a skin bruise has a purple color that transitions over time to green and yellow as heme is oxidized and sequentially converted to biliverdin and bilirubin.

Transport and metabolism of bilirubin

Although molecular diagrams of bilirubin suggest that it should be water soluble, the opposite is true. In brief, it folds in on itself forming intramolecular hydrogen bonds, resulting in a high level of hydrophobicity [1]. Within the circulation, bilirubin is solubilized by virtue of high-affinity binding to albumin, and within cells, it is solubilized by binding to cytosolic proteins, especially the glutathione S-transferases (GSTs) to which it binds tightly as a nonsubstrate ligand.

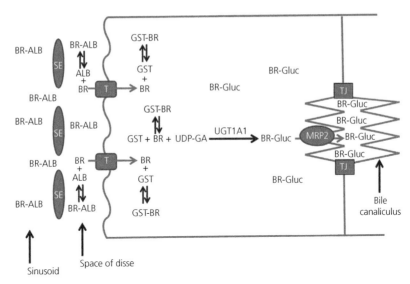

Figure 12.2 Schematic diagram of the liver as it relates to bilirubin transport and metabolism: bilirubin has very low aqueous solubility and circulates in the blood stream bound tightly to albumin. Fenestrations in the sinusoidal endothelium (SE) permit the albumin–bilirubin complex to enter the space of Disse and come into proximity of hepatocyte microvilli that contain a bilirubin transporter (T) that facilitates entry into the hepatocyte of the unbound bilirubin that is in equilibrium with albumin-bound bilirubin. Within the hepatocyte, bilirubin binds to GSTs as a nonsubstrate ligand and is conjugated with glucuronic acid in a reaction catalyzed by the enzyme UGT1A1 and requiring UDP-GA [7]. Conjugation of bilirubin with glucuronic acid renders it water soluble, and it is then pumped out of the cell into the bile canalicular space by an ATP-dependent pump (MRP2). The bile canaliculus represents a specialized area of the hepatocyte plasma membrane. It is isolated from the sinusoidal plasma membrane by junctional complexes including tight junctions (TJ).

After formation in reticuloendothelial cells, bilirubin is released into the circulation where it complexes rapidly with albumin. Under normal conditions, little if any bilirubin enters nonhepatic tissues. In contrast, in a single pass through the liver, as much as 30% of bilirubin is extracted from its albumin carrier and enters hepatocytes. Although some research had suggested that albumin binds to a receptor on the hepatocyte surface facilitating bilirubin release, subsequent studies have not substantiated this hypothesis [3]. It is thought that a small free fraction of bilirubin interacts directly with a transporter on the hepatocyte surface and that reestablishment of the binding equilibrium provides a continuous unbound fraction of bilirubin that is available for transport into hepatocytes.

Circulating bilirubin–albumin complexes are able to pass through fenestrations in the hepatic sinusoidal endothelium and enter the space of Disse, an extracellular, extravascular space unique to the liver that constitutes approximately 30% of its extracellular volume (Figure 12.2) [4]. This geometry permits the small fraction of unbound bilirubin to interact directly with a specific transport protein on the hepatocyte surface that facilitates its entry into the cell where it subsequently binds to GSTs, as noted previously. Although studies have indicated that bilirubin transport by hepatocytes has characteristics of a protein-mediated process, the identity of the transporter remains elusive and is a subject of continued investigation [5, 6].

Within the hepatocyte, bilirubin is conjugated with glucuronic acid in a reaction catalyzed by the enzyme UDP-glucuronosyl transferase isoform 1A1 (UGT1A1) and requiring UDP-glucuronic acid (UDP-GA) [7]. Interestingly, this enzyme is located in the endoplasmic reticulum. There is little known about the mechanisms that allow bilirubin to move in and out of this intracellular organelle. Conjugation of bilirubin with glucuronic acid renders it water soluble because after conjugation it is no longer able to form intramolecular hydrogen bonds. Three familial nonhemolytic disorders characterized by unconjugated hyperbilirubinemia all have defects of the UGT1A1 molecule and differ in the level of residual enzyme activity. Crigler–Najjar syndrome type I has the greatest reduction of enzyme activity with levels barely, if even, detectable. Although all other aspects of liver function are normal, if left untreated, affected individuals will develop kernicterus and usually die during infancy. As just a small amount of enzyme activity can maintain bilirubin below toxic levels, this disorder has served as an impetus to develop novel treatments including gene therapy and hepatocyte transplantation. There is usually sufficient UGT1A1 activity in patients with Crigler–Najjar syndrome type II to keep serum bilirubin below toxic levels, although it can be quite elevated. On very rare occasions, intercurrent illness such as influenza can result in abrupt elevation of unconjugated bilirubin in affected patients and consequent neurologic injury [8]. In contrast to the two Crigler–Najjar syndromes, Gilbert syndrome is a common disorder that is found in at least 5% of the population at large. It too is associated with reduced activity of UGT1A1, although to a more modest degree, resulting in bilirubin levels generally being less than 3.0 mg/dl. Interestingly, the coding region for UGT1A1 is usually normal in these patients who instead have mutations in the gene's promoter region that can result in reduced transcription of the UGT1A1 gene and subsequent reduced expression of the enzyme. Although patients with Gilbert syndrome are healthy, they have been described as having reduced metabolism of some drugs that are normally glucuronidated by the liver, especially an active metabolite of the chemotherapeutic agent irinotecan.

After normal conjugation with glucuronic acid, bilirubin is pumped out of the cell into the bile canaliculus by an ATP-dependent pump termed the multi-drug resistance associated protein 2 (MRP2), which is localized to the canalicular plasma membrane of the hepatocyte [9]. Patients with defects in this pump have the Dubin–Johnson syndrome, an abnormality that has been described in populations throughout the world, most commonly in Iranian Jews in whom the frequency of the disorder approaches 1:1200 [10]. Total serum bilirubin concentrations in affected individuals usually range between 2 and 5 mg/dl, although levels within the normal range or as high as 20 mg/dl can be seen. These patients have no evidence of cholestasis, and serum alkaline phosphatase and bile acid levels are normal. Rotor syndrome is a rare abnormality phenotypically similar to Dubin–Johnson syndrome that is caused by simultaneous mutations in two sinusoidal plasma membrane transporters, OATP1B1 and OATP1B3, which normally take up conjugated bilirubin from the blood [11]. A novel mechanism has been suggested whereby conjugated bilirubin produced in hepatocytes is secreted back into the circulation and subjected to reuptake, mediated by OATP1B1 and OATP1B3. When these proteins are defective, the reuptake mechanism is perturbed, and conjugated hyperbilirubinemia develops.

Extrahepatic fate of excreted bilirubin

Once excreted into the bile, conjugated bilirubin moves through the small intestine with little absorption or biotransformation. Upon entering the colon, however, a fraction is deconjugated by bacterial β-glucuronidase, and this unconjugated bilirubin can be reabsorbed, extracted from the portal circulation by hepatocytes, reconjugated, and re-excreted [12]. This enterohepatic cycle is normally of little clinical importance, but its interruption with sequestering agents can be therapeutic in some instances of hyperbilirubinemia. Other bacterial enzymes in the colon can degrade bilirubin to colorless compounds including urobilinogen. Urobilinogen is water soluble and can be absorbed and re-excreted by the liver as well as the kidney. Conditions associated with increased bilirubin production (e.g., hemolysis) or reduced hepatic elimination of bilirubin can be associated with increased urinary excretion of urobilinogen, which is often measured by routine dipstick analysis. Determination of urinary urobilinogen is usually not diagnostically useful, except when it is absent in the face of substantial jaundice. This combination of findings can signify complete obstruction of bile flow such that bilirubin is not excreted into the intestine and consequently urobilinogen is not produced. As noted in the preceding text, unconjugated bilirubin is not water soluble. As a rule of thumb, it will never appear in urine, in contrast to urinary excretion of conjugated bilirubin even with low circulating levels.

Clinical laboratory determination of serum bilirubin

Any review of bilirubin should include consideration of how it is measured in the clinical chemistry laboratory. Although sophisticated procedures exist to very accurately determine levels of bilirubin and its conjugates in blood, these are not used routinely, due to considerations of cost and time. Most laboratories use an assay in which bilirubin reacts with a diazo reagent, forming a colored compound.

Unconjugated bilirubin reacts slowly with the agent, while conjugated bilirubin reacts rapidly. Direct-reacting bilirubin, that is, that portion of the total bilirubin that forms a colored diazo compound within 1 m, is therefore taken as a measure of the serum conjugated bilirubin content. Total bilirubin is determined after addition of an accelerant, for example, ethanol, that causes unconjugated bilirubin to also react quickly with the diazo agent. The indirect bilirubin is determined (indirectly) by subtracting the direct-reacting fraction from the total bilirubin and is used as a measure of unconjugated bilirubin. It is not surprising that this assay produces estimates that are somewhat inaccurate [13, 14]. For example, diazo assay of a solution of pure unconjugated bilirubin would show that 15–20% was direct-reacting even in the absence of an accelerant. As elevated conjugated bilirubin in the serum can often signify hepatobiliary dysfunction, a laboratory report of mildly elevated direct-reacting bilirubin should cause concern. Because conjugated bilirubin, even at low levels, is readily excreted in the urine, dipstick analysis of urine for bilirubin in this situation can resolve any uncertainty.

The one situation in which elevated direct-reacting bilirubin is not reflected in bilirubin urinary excretion is the presence of δ-bilirubin in the circulation [15]. This is formed in the presence of prolonged conjugated hyperbilirubinemia and represents covalent bilirubin attachment to albumin. This albumin-attached bilirubin reacts quickly with diazo reagent (direct-reacting) but is not filtered by the kidney and does not appear in urine. It disappears slowly from the circulation commensurate with turnover of albumin (half-life of 20 days). δ-bilirubin can be responsible for slow clearance of direct-reacting bilirubin following reversal of long-standing cholestasis such as seen after decompression of biliary obstruction or with resolution of cholestatic hepatitis. At present, there is no routine assay for δ-bilirubin.

Evaluation of the patient with hyperbilirubinemia

Jaundice is a diagnosis made on physical examination that signifies a total bilirubin level of at least 2.5–3.0 mg/dl (Table 12.1). Detection of jaundice is affected by variable conditions that include ambient light and skin and scleral coloring. The lower limit of normal for serum bilirubin is approximately 1.0–1.4 mg/dl, depending on the particular assay used by the clinical laboratory. Thus, patients can have hyperbilirubinemia but not jaundice. It should be emphasized that the clinical implications of hyperbilirubinemia are identical whether or not the patient has jaundice. In most hepatobiliary disorders, with the exception of some familial syndromes (mentioned earlier), hyperbilirubinemia is due to elevated levels of unconjugated and conjugated bilirubin. Although it is tempting to attribute clinical importance to the ratio of the two, this is inaccurate and not helpful in differential diagnosis. Conjugated bilirubin is cleared by the kidney, and its accumulation in serum is determined by both hepatic and renal function. In cases of liver dysfunction

Table 12.1 Comparison of inheritable disorders characterized by unconjugated or conjugated hyperbilirubinemia.

	Total serum bilirubin (mg/dl)	Incidence	Morbidity	Inheritance	Liver morphology	Molecular defect
Unconjugated hyperbilirubinemias						
Crigler–Najjar I	20–50	Rare (<1:1 000 000)	Kernicterus and death in infancy if untreated	Autosomal recessive	Normal	Markedly reduced UGT1A1 activity
Crigler–Najjar II	3–15	Uncommon	Usually cosmetic but rarely late-onset kernicterus can occur with intercurrent illness	Autosomal recessive	Normal	UGT1A1 activity reduced by 90%
Gilbert	2–3.5	Common (>5%)	None	Autosomal recessive and dominant forms	Normal	UGT1A1 activity reduced by 50–90%
Conjugated hyperbilirubinemias						
Dubin–Johnson	2–5	Uncommon	None	Autosomal recessive	Black pigment, otherwise normal	Mutated MRP2
Rotor	2–5	Rare (<1:1 000 000)	None	Autosomal recessive	Normal	Mutations in OATP1B1 and OATP1B3

in the face of renal failure, total bilirubin levels in the circulation can be very high (e.g., >40 mg/dl) due to loss of this renal "overflow" mechanism. In general, mixed conjugated and unconjugated hyperbilirubinemia accompanied by other abnormalities of routine liver tests (e.g., alanine aminotransferase elevation) signifies an acquired hepatobiliary disorder that needs further evaluation as to cause. In these circumstances, the hyperbilirubinemia itself is a clinical sign of liver dysfunction. Unconjugated hyperbilirubinemia is diagnosed when total serum bilirubin is elevated due to elevated unconjugated bilirubin. Although, as discussed previously, the clinical laboratory may report elevated direct-reacting bilirubin, there will be no bilirubin in the urine. The finding of unconjugated hyperbilirubinemia implies increased bilirubin production (e.g., hemolysis) or reduced uptake or conjugation by hepatocytes (e.g., Gilbert syndrome). There have been no disorders with hyperbilirubinemia that have been conclusively attributed to dysfunction of the uptake mechanism for bilirubin, although several drugs might compete with bilirubin for uptake and have been associated with transient mild hyperbilirubinemia [16, 17].

Multiple choice questions

1 A 20-year-old woman presents to the emergency department with vomiting and diarrhea that started 12 h previously. On physical examination, she is afebrile but appears mildly dehydrated with icteric sclerae. Examination of the abdomen reveals hyperactive bowel sounds without enlargement or tenderness of the liver or spleen. Laboratory examination is notable for bilirubin of 3.5/0.2 mg/dl (total/direct), normal white blood count and hematocrit, and normal liver function tests (ALT, AST, alkaline phosphatase). Which one of the following diagnoses is the most likely cause of her jaundice?
   A Acute viral hepatitis
   B Dubin–Johnson syndrome
   C Acute cholecystitis
   D Gilbert syndrome
   E Common bile duct obstruction
2 A 53-year-old man presents with jaundice and is found to have a large mass in the head of the pancreas. Laboratory examination shows that his serum bilirubin is 23/12 mg/dl (total/direct). Urinalysis is remarkable for 4+ bilirubin and absent urobilinogen. Which one of the following statements concerning this patient is most likely true?
   A He is at risk of developing kernicterus.
   B He has complete bile duct obstruction.
   C The bilirubin in his urine is mostly unconjugated.
   D His liver cannot synthesize urobilinogen because of an enzyme deficiency.
   E His sclerae will not be yellow because his kidneys are excreting so much bilirubin.
3 A 21-year-old woman comes in for a routine physical examination and is found to have scleral icterus. She has no complaints, and the rest of her physical exam is unremarkably normal. She recently started taking oral contraceptives. She is on no other medications. Laboratory examination shows normal liver function tests including ALT, AST, and alkaline phosphatase. Her serum bilirubin is 4.2/3.6 mg/dl (total/direct), and dipstick analysis of her urine shows 3+ bilirubin. Which one of the following statements concerning this patient is most likely true?

    A Gallstones must be considered as a highly likely cause of her jaundice.

    B Her laboratory values are most compatible with chronic hemolysis.

    C She has developed a cholestatic reaction from the oral contraceptives.

    D She has Dubin–Johnson syndrome.

    E She needs to be evaluated for cholestatic hepatitis.

4 A newborn baby has extreme elevations of the serum indirect bilirubin, and there is concern about kernicterus. The baby is treated with phototherapy. The most likely enzyme deficiency in this is baby is?

    A Aldolase B

    B Uroporphyrinogen decarboxylase

    C Glucose 6-phosphatase

    D Uridine diphosphate-glucuronosyl transferase

    E Galactose-1-phosphate uridyltransferase

References

1 Wolkoff, A.W., and Berk, P.D. (2012) Bilirubin metabolism and jaundice, in *Schiff's Diseases of the Liver*, 11th edn (eds E.R. Schiff, W.C. Maddrey and M.F. Sorrell), Wiley, Hoboken, pp. 120–151.

2 Leffler, C.W., Parfenova, H. and Jaggar, J.H. (2011) Carbon monoxide as an endogenous vascular modulator. *American Journal of Physiology. Heart and Circulatory Physiology*, **301**, H1–H11.

3 Stollman, Y.R., Gartner, U., Theilmann, L. *et al.* (1983) Hepatic bilirubin uptake in the isolated perfused rat liver is not facilitated by albumin binding. *Journal of Clinical* Investigation, **72**, 718–723.

4 Grisham, J.W., Nopanitaya, W., Compagno, J. and Nagel, A.E. (1975) Scanning electron microscopy of normal rat liver: the surface structure of its cells and tissue components. *American Journal of Anatomy*, **144**, 295–321.

5 Wang, P., Kim, R.B., Chowdhury, J.R. and Wolkoff, A.W. (2003) The human organic anion transport protein SLC21A6 is not sufficient for bilirubin transport. *Journal of Biological Chemistry*, **278**, 20695–20699.

6 Wolkoff, A.W. (2012) Mechanisms of hepatocyte organic anion transport, in *Physiology of the Gastrointestinal Tract*, 5th edn (eds L.R. Johnson, F.K. Ghishan, J.D. Kaunitz *et al.*), Academic Press, San Diego, pp. 1485–1506.

7 Strassburg, C.P., Lankisch, T.O., Manns, M.P. and Ehmer, U. (2008) Family 1 uridine-5'-diphosphate glucuronosyltransferases (UGT1A): from Gilbert's syndrome to genetic organization and variability. *Archives of Toxicology*, **82**, 415–433.

8 Gordon, E.R., Shaffer, E.A. and Sass-Kortsak, A. (1976) Bilirubin secretion and conjugation in the Crigler-Najjar syndrome type II. *Gastroenterology*, **70**, 761–765.

9 Nies, A.T. and Keppler, D. (2007) The apical conjugate efflux pump ABCC2 (MRP2). *Pflügers Archiv – European Journal of Physiology*, **453**, 643–659.

10 Shani, M., Seligsohn, U., Gilon, E. *et al.* (1970) Dubin-Johnson syndrome in Israel. I. Clinical, laboratory, and genetic aspects of 101 cases. *Quarterly Journal of Medicine*, **39**, 549–567.

11 van de Steg, E., Stranecky, V., Hartmannova, H. *et al.* (2012) Complete OATP1B1 and OATP1B3 deficiency causes human Rotor syndrome by interrupting conjugated bilirubin reuptake into the liver. *Journal of Clinical Investigation*, **122**, 519–528.

12 Poland, R.L. and Odell, G.B. (1971) Physiologic jaundice: the enterohepatic circulation of bilirubin. *New England Journal of Medicine*, **284**, 1–6.

13 Lott, J.A. and Doumas, B.T. (1993) "Direct" and total bilirubin tests: contemporary problems. *Clinical Chemistry*, **39**, 641–647.

14 Doumas, B.T. and Eckfeldt, J.H. (1996) Errors in measurement of total bilirubin: a perennial problem. *Clinical Chemistry*, **42**, 845–848.

15 Doumas, B.T., Wu, T.W. and Jendrzejczak, B. (1987) Delta bilirubin: absorption spectra, molar absorptivity, and reactivity in the diazo reaction. *Clinical Chemistry*, **33**, 769–774.

16 Acocella, G., Nicolis, F.B. and Tenconi, L.T. (1965) The effect of an intravenous infusion of rifamycin SV on the excretion of bilirubin, bromsulphalein, and indocyanine green in man. *Gastroenterology*, **49**, 521–530.

17 Kenwright, S. and Levi, A.J. (1974) Sites of competition in the selective hepatic uptake of rifamycin-SV, flavaspidic acid, bilirubin, and bromsulphthalein. *Gut*, **15**, 220–226.

Answers

1 D
2 B
3 D
4 D

Index

Note: Page numbers in *italics* refer to Figures; those in **bold** to Tables.

Gastrointestinal Anatomy and Physiology: The Essentials, First Edition. Edited by John F. Reinus and Douglas Simon.
© 2014 John Wiley & Sons, Ltd. Published 2014 by John Wiley & Sons, Ltd.
www.wiley.com/go/reinus/gastro/anatomy

Printed and bound by CPI Group (UK) Ltd, Croydon, CR0 4YY

27/10/2024

14580144-0002